Bacteria as Plant Pathogens

Dr Billing was formerly Research Pathologist at the East Malling Research Station. She had previously been Lecturer in Microbiology at the University of Reading.

Aspects of Microbiology 14

Bacteria as Plant Pathogens

Eve Billing

VNR UK **Van Nostrand Reinhold (UK) Co. Ltd**

First published in 1987 by
Van Nostrand Reinhold (UK) Co. Ltd
Molly Millars Lane, Wokingham, Berkshire, England

Typeset in Times 9 on 10pt by
Colset Private Ltd, Singapore

Printed and bound in Hong Kong

British Library Cataloguing in Publication Data
Billing, Eve
Bacteria as plant pathogens. — (Aspects of microbiology; 14).
1. Bacteria, Phytopathogenic
I. Title II. Series
581.2'322 QR351

ISBN 0-278-00010-X
(ISSN 0266-6642)

Contents

Preface

This book aims to provide an introduction to plant pathogenic bacteria. Though written primarily for undergraduate microbiology students the needs of postgraduates and people in related disciplines have also been considered, for example mammalian pathologists, plant pathologists turning from fungal to bacterial diseases in their research, and biochemists and geneticists who may want to gain a broader view of bacterial plant pathogens.

Since the interaction of bacteria with plants is very much a multidisciplinary topic, problems of communication are common, so terminology has been kept as simple as possible. Specialist terms, where they must be used, are defined and dual meanings discussed. The number of publications by specialists for specialists in this area is rapidly increasing and can leave some readers with the mistaken impression that the subject is more complex than it really is, or that particular findings are applicable to pathogens other than the ones studied.

The book makes few assumptions about prior knowledge and aims to provide enough basic information to equip the reader to follow specialist topics in further depth without undue difficulty. However, there is also a rounded account for those that desire it, avoiding undue speculation which might cloud issues where clear understanding remains elusive.

Taxonomy and nomenclature are covered briefly to give guidance on current usage. To simplify discussion, the pathogens have been divided into three main groups based on the major symptoms produced: necrosis, tissue maceration and gall induction. There is, however, some overlap between the groups, particularly in the case of vascular wilt pathogens.

The plants as hosts and the bacteria as pathogens are first considered separately. The importance of water potential in both plant and bacterial physiology is emphasized. There follows a description of bacterial products that appear to be of particular significance in plant pathogenicity.

Interactions between the pathogen and the host at the molecular and cellular levels are discussed in detail, starting with pathogen entry into plant tissues and then considering the ways in which the plant succeeds or fails in countering invasion. The nature of host specificity is considered. The hypersensitive reaction in plants is described and distinguished from that in mammals where, unfortunately and confusingly, the same term is used to describe certain immune responses.

The genetics of the plant-pathogen interaction is then considered. The few examples of current findings are described with full awareness that this is the area, alongside the investigation of underlying mechanisms of plant pathogen interactions, where advances may be rapid.

The book ends on the subject of epidemiology and control, noting the special difficulties encountered in the control of bacterial diseases in plants compared with those in mammals and with fungal plant diseases.

Rather than quote names of all who have helped me on specialist topics (most of their names appear in the suggestions for further reading), I dedicate this book to them, to all my teachers and fellow enthusiasts who in the past kept my mind stimulated on these matters, and to any readers who use this book as a base for the pursuit of further knowledge. I am particularly grateful to R. M. Cooper and J. W. Mansfield who allowed me to see unpublished manuscripts and to the Series editors for valuable comment and constructive criticism.

EVE BILLING

1 Introduction

For many years, the study of plant pathogenic bacteria was the province of a small group of biologists. Since the 1970s interest has broadened due largely to developments in immunological techniques and in molecular biology and to the ease with which plant pathogenic bacteria can be manipulated genetically compared with their fungal counterparts.

In the past, because of their greater importance in terms of crop losses, plant pathologists concentrated on fungal and viral diseases, rather than on bacterial ones. In contrast, animal and human pathologists devoted most attention to bacterial and viral diseases. Bacteriologists were drawn more often towards the study of mammalian rather than plant pathogens and few had a good basic understanding of or interest in plant biology. Similarly, though well equipped to study fungi, plant pathologists often lacked the skills necessary to study bacteria.

Divergence of interests often leads to barriers of communication between disciplines and only a few biologists have managed to move happily between mammalian and plant pathology and benefit fully from the resultant cross feeding. Cross-disciplinary approaches are now breaking such barriers. Some, however, remain and new ones may appear if molecular biologists and pathologists do not keep in close touch so that the latter can appreciate and use the contributions that molecular biologists can make towards understanding pathogenic processes and disease control.

This book cannot cover all aspects of interdisciplinary communication but, where possible, mammalian and plant systems will be compared, similarities and differences between fungal and bacterial plant pathogens noted, and the current impact of molecular biology described. Molecular biology is a rapidly expanding field so only an outline of present trends will be possible.

Guidance on further reading is provided at the end of each chapter, and a bibliography on p. 75 extends the area of study.

Economic importance

Crop losses caused by bacterial diseases are difficult to assess (Garrett in Rhodes-Roberts and Skinner, 1982; Deacon in *Aspects* 7, 1983 *see* Bibliography). Bacterial diseases are generally of lower economic importance than diseases caused by fungi and viruses. However, in some cases, a crop which should be profitable cannot be grown because a bacterial pathogen is too destructive in too many seasons. Examples include bacterial wilt (*Pseudomonas solanacearum*) of potato, tomato and other crops and fire blight (*Erwinia amylovora*) of pears. Of the staple food crops, severe losses in some years have been reported for rice (*Xanthomonas campestris* pv. *oryzae*), wheat (*Pseudomonas syringae*), soya bean (*P. syringae* pv. *glycinea*), cassava (*P.s.* pv. *manihotis*) and potato (*Erwinia carotovora*); in the last case, losses are mainly from storage rots and can be great. The economic importance of bacterial diseases is greater in subtropical than in temperate climates.

History of the study of bacterial plant pathogens

The first plant disease suspected of being caused by bacteria was fire blight (*E. amylovora*), a serious necrotic disease of pear and apple trees in USA at the time. T. J. Burrill was convinced of its bacterial origin as early as 1878 but it was not until 1885 that J. C. Arthur used pure cultures to provide convincing proof. During the same period various human and animal bacterial diseases were first described. In 1920, Erwin F. Smith gave a detailed account of 14 bacterial plant diseases and provided notes on others in a comprehensive textbook illustrated with many photomicrographs of diseased plant tissue and the bacterial pathogens. No comparable book has been published since.

In books published between 1948 and 1961, W.J. Dowson and C. Stapp helped to sustain interest in the subject. Charlotte Elliott, in 1951, wrote a comprehensive *Manual of Bacterial Plant Pathogens* listing synonyms, characteristics of the bacteria in laboratory tests, host range, symptoms, geographical distribution, control methods and references (see Bradbury, 1986). The number of newly described species became unwieldy because whenever a disease was described for a new host a new species was named. By 1957 in *Bergey's Manual of Determinative Bacteriology* there were 50 species in the genus *Xanthomonas* alone.

The 1960s showed a general upsurge of interest in bacterial taxonomy based at first on cultural, nutritional and biochemical characters and often applying techniques of numerical taxonomy. By the 1970s, data on DNA, RNA and protein homology were used and, in the 1980s, fatty acid profiles. It is unfortunate that bacterial plant pathogens and other plant-associated bacteria are sometimes ignored in taxonomic studies. By the 1980s, in the interests of cross-disciplinary communication, there was a move towards grouping like organisms and away from a multiplicity of species in all branches of bacteriology. As a result, in 1980 the Judicial Commission of the International Committee of Systematic Bacteriology recognized only five *Xanthomonas* species; many of the old species were classed as *pathovars*. The merits of these decisions and problems posed by rigid taxonomic rules lie outside the scope of this book, but the need remains to group like bacteria and to distinguish those that produce distinct diseases. No doubt debate, sometimes acrimonious, will continue on what constitutes a species and what is in the best interests of communication within and between disciplines.

In the 1970s, there was an explosion of interest in fundamental studies on plant pathogenic bacteria. This stemmed largely from a report that the factor which induced gall formation could be transferred from a pathogenic to a non-pathogenic strain of *Agrobacterium tumefaciens*. By the mid-1970s research workers in several laboratories had demonstrated that genes for tumour induction by *Agrobacterium* were located on a large plasmid. It appeared that the plasmid could be used as a vector for the introduction of foreign DNA into plants susceptible to infection by *A. tumefaciens*. Crown gall is not however, typical of other diseases as it induces host cell and tissue proliferation, not cell death.

Research on bacterial diseases where there is host cell and tissue death has also continued at an increased pace. A powerful stimulus has been the improvements in electron microscopy and new serological techniques, including the use of ELISA and fluorescent and monoclonal antibodies. There have also been advances in understanding the nature and properties of some of the low-molecular-weight toxins and cellular interactions between host plants and bacteria. Binding of bacteria to cell surfaces has received much attention. Glycoproteins were once thought to have a major role in specific adhesion but increased understanding of the influence of charge and hydrophobicity on interacting molecules and on non-specific binding changed the emphasis of this work. These facets and their relationship to host resistance, the hypersensitive reaction and the role of extracellular polysaccharides in virulence are discussed in Chapters 3 and 4. Modern techniques and genetic approaches (see Chapter 5) should lead within the next decade to improved understanding of the underlying mechanisms of pathogenesis.

Major types of disease

Blights and cankers These start as local areas of cell death (necrosis) and may show as leaf, pod or fruit spots or blossom death (blights) or stem lesions (cankers). The disease may remain localized or become systemic and spread through the plant. These diseases have dramatic names such as blast, black arm and wild fire. Pathogens causing necrosis will be called *necrogens* here. The precise cause of cell death is uncertain.

Vascular wilts This term is used for diseases where xylem vessels are invaded by necrogenic pathogens and wilting is the most obvious symptom. Extracellular polysaccharides often have a role in disease development but cell wall degrading enzymes and alterations in plant growth regulator balance may also be involved.

Soft rots These occur when there is host cell separation (maceration) leading to tissue collapse; the dead tissue remains soft and moist. Pathogens causing these diseases will be called *macergens* here. This last term is not in general use and it not suggested that it should be widely adopted outside the context of this book. Some readers will prefer the terms *macerators* or *soft rotters*.

Table 1 Characteristics of the major types of bacterial disease

Disease type induced[a]	Compatibility response	Incompatibility response	Host range
Necrotic leaf spot and stem canker (*necrogen*)	Delayed plant cell death (necrosis)	Rapid plant cell death (HR)	Usually narrow
Progressive soft rot in advance of pathogen (*macergen*)	Tissue destruction (maceration)	None at low doses	Often wide
Gall formation; tissue shoot or root proliferation (*oncogen*)	Uncontrolled cell division (gall formation)	None (rare exceptions)	Often wide

[a] Pathogen group in parenthesis. Some pathogens have properties of more than one group. Some necrogens also induce wilting. Ice nucleation during frosts may cause necrosis.

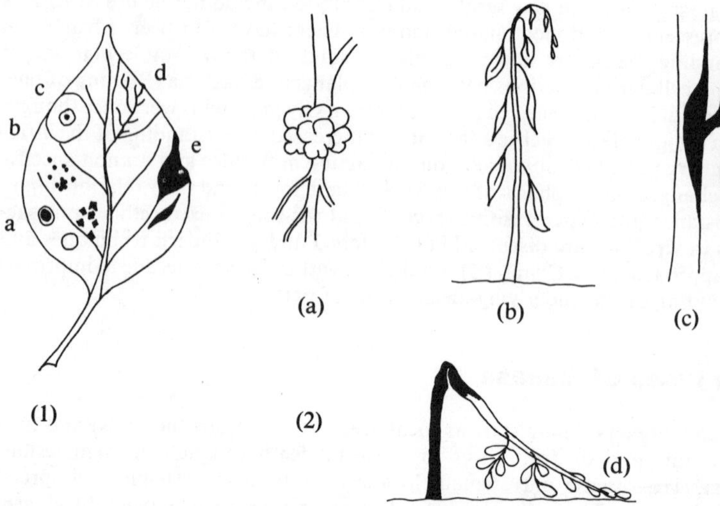

Fig. 1 Some characteristic symptoms produced by plant pathogenic bacteria. (1) Leaf lesions (a) 'shot hole' of cherry *Pseudomonas syringae* pv. *morsprunorum* – the necrotic lesions drop out; (b) small and angular necrotic spots (some *P. syringae* and *Xanthomonas campestris* pathovars); (c) necrotic spot surrounded by a water-soaked area and a large chlorotic halo (halo blight, *P. s.* pv. *phaseolicola*); (d) black veins following hydathode invasion (black rot of crucifers, *X. c.* pv. *campestris*); (e) large necrotic areas (*Corynebacterium michiganense* pv. *michiganense*). (2) Stem lesions (a) crown gall (*Agrobacterium tumefaciens*); (b) vascular wilt (*Pseudomonas solanacearum*); (c) necrosis, wilt and stem canker (fire blight, *Erwinia amylovora*). (d) stem rot (black leg, *Erwinia carotovora* pv. *atroseptica*).

Galls These form as a result of host cell proliferation resulting in cancer-like tissue growth or root, stem or leaf proliferation. The pathogens concerned will be called *oncogens* (tumour-causing) here.

Different types of pathogen

In writing this book it seemed more useful to distinguish pathogens on the basis of the symptoms they produce than on their nutritional strategy, which is usual with fungi (see Chapter 2). In particular, it was essential to distinguish clearly between necrogenic and macergenic *Erwinia* and *Pseudomonas* spp., for example, between *E. amylovora* and *E. carotovora* and between *P. syringae* and *P. marginalis* (Table 2). However, not all pathogens fall clearly into a single group.

Both plants and animals are in constant contact with a wide range of bacteria yet only a very small proportion of these bacteria cause serious disease. When host resistance is reduced (for example by mechanical, nutritional or environmental stress), normally harmless bacteria may induce disease; they are referred to as *opportunistic pathogens*. It is only among these bacteria that there sometimes

Table 2 Some representative plant pathogenic bacteria

Genus	Species, pathovar[a]	Disease[b]
Gram negative		
Agrobacterium	*tumefaciens*	Crown gall
Erwinia	*amylovora*	Fire blight (pear)
	carotovora pv. *carotovora*	Soft rots
	pv. *atroseptica*	Black leg (potato)
	chrysanthemi	Soft rots
	stewartii	Bacterial wilt (maize)
Pseudomonas	*marginalis*	Soft rots
	syringae pv. *syringae*	Various
	pv. *phaseolicola*	Halo blight (bean)
	pv. *tabaci*	Wild fire (tobacco)
	pv. *savastanoi*	Olive knot
	solanacearum (3 races)	Bacterial wilt
Xanthomonas	*campestris* pv. *campestris*	Black rot (crucifers)
	pv. *phaseoli*	Common blight (bean)
	malvacearum	Black arm (cotton)
	albilineans	Leaf scald (sugar cane)
Gram positive		
Corynebacterium fascians (*Rhodobacterium*)		Leafy gall
Corynebacterium michiganense (*Clavibacter*)	pv. *michiganense*	Bacterial canker (tomato)
	pv. *insidiosum*	Bacterial wilt (lucerne)
	pv. *sepedonicum*	Ring rot (potato)
Corynebacterium flaccumfaciens (*Curtobacterium*)	pv. *flaccumfaciens*	Bacterial wilt (bean)

[a] Throughout this book the following abbreviations will be used. For pathovars of *E. carotovora*, *P. syringae*, *X. campestris* and *C. michiganense*: *E. c.*, *P. s.*, *X. c.* and *C. m.* respectively. For example *E. c. atroseptica*, *P. s. phaseolicola*, *X. c. malvacearum* and *C. m. sepedonicum*. Provided there is no risk of ambiguity, only the initial of the generic name will be used. (Such extreme abbreviation is not acceptable in all scientific publications.)

[b] Examples of necrogens: *P. syringae* and *X. campestris* pvs, *P. solanacearum*; macergens: *E. carotovora*, *E. chrysanthemi*, *P. marginalis*; oncogens: *A. tumefaciens*, *C. fascians*. Some of the remaining species are difficult to allocate to a single group.

appears to be overlap between mammalian and plant pathogens. Such cases need to be examined critically. Those associated with plant disease may differ in some character, such as pectic enzyme production, from those associated with mammalian disease, though they appear to belong to the same species. It is not easy to judge how far plant-associated bacteria pose a real risk to humans and animals. Opportunistic plant pathogens receive brief mention elsewhere in the book but the main concern is with pathogens that cause disease in healthy plants.

Fastidious pathogenic prokaryotes

This book concentrates on nutritionally non-exacting pathogens on which studies on host-pathogen relationships at the molecular level are currently focused. Brief mention must be made, however, of the small, fastidious prokaryotes (FP). As few of these have been cultured, much work is still at the descriptive rather than the analytical stage. The diversity of this group also makes simple generalizations difficult. For further information see Behncken in Fahy and Persley (1983); Bové (1984); Daniels in Rhodes-Roberts and Skinner (1982); Rosenberger in Mount and Lacey (1982).

The FP group contains small rod-shaped bacteria (usually less than 0.5 μm diameter) whose taxonomic position is unclear. Some are referred to as rickettsia-like bacteria (RLB) but they do not closely resemble rickettsia from animal sources. A few have been cultivated on complex media.

MLOs

Quite distinct are the wall-free mollicutes commonly referred to as *mycoplasma*-like organisms (MLO). They include the saprophyte *Acholeplasma*, which is found in association with both plants and animals, and pathogens which have been observed in plant tissue but have not yet been cultured; they were previously mistaken for viruses. Also wall-free are the *Spiroplasma* which form helical filaments and are motile. Some have been cultured so they are the best understood group.

The majority of RLB and MLO exclusively colonize xylem vessels or phloem seive tubes and are transmitted only by sucking insects such as leaf hoppers or by grafting during plant propagation. RLB tend to multiply only in the foregut of insects but some MLO multiply and circulate in insect tissue and eventually infect salivary glands. Some of the spiroplasmas are pathogenic for their insect vectors. Disease is transmitted during feeding so it is not surprising that spiroplasmas are sometimes isolated from parts of healthy plants, such as blossoms, commonly visited by insects. Many FP have a wide host range but this will to some extent be controlled by their insect vectors.

RLB may be phloem- or xylem-limited or not restricted to a particular host tissue. Most MLO are phloem-limited; absence of a rigid cell wall no doubt aids their movement through seive plates. The high osmotic pressure of seive tube contents helps to maintain MLO cell integrity. MLO appear to be associated most commonly with young leaves, where the turnover of nutrients is high.

Symptoms produced in the host plant by RLB and MLO vary widely and include yellowing, stunting, leaf distortion and shoot proliferation. Such symptoms may be attributable to a reduction in the availability of nutrients to host tissue, impaired water flow and disturbance of growth regulator balance. Toxins might have a role in some cases but, in general, pathogenic strategies are poorly understood.

Spiroplasmas that can be cultured are being studied in depth; a plasmid has been cloned and a spiroplasma gene is expressed in *Escherichia coli*. Plant viral DNA appears to be a possible vector for cloning spiroplasma genes. Spiroplasmas invade their insect vectors making this a particularly fascinating area for research because host-parasite interactions can be studied in both plant and insect.

Taxonomy and nomenclature

The taxonomy of plant pathogenic bacteria has been a topic for considerable debate and current approaches are not universally approved (Schaad in Mount and Lacey, 1982). Nevertheless, they form a good basis for communication between disciplines and the issues need not be a cause for concern here. Plant pathogens present particular problems because there are many different host plants of economic importance and, in the case of necrogens, often a high degree of host specificity. This led in the past to the cumbersome multiplicity of pathogen species. Modern taxonomic methods, including protein and fatty acid profiles, are helping to improve groupings of like bacteria and to distinguish between bacteria causing diseases on different hosts. The dilemma is the need for pathologists to recognize each specific pathogen so that risk of spread of disease, especially between countries, can be reduced to a minimum as against the scientific value of grouping similar organisms. For communication the name of the pathogen should, ideally, reflect both.

Once generic and specific names are agreed, the pathologist may need to identify subgroups of strains isolated from particular cases of a disease, especially where different hosts are affected. Subgroups may be based primarily on host specificity and the term *pathovar* (pv.) is now widely used (Dye *et al.*, 1980; Moffett and Dye in Fahy and Persley, 1983). In *P. solanacearum* the term *race* is applied but this term is also used for different strains of a pathovar which infect different cultivars of a host species (see Chapter 5). Because of the practical difficulties of performing host-range tests, cultural, biochemical, serological and phage and bacteriocin sensitivity tests are used in attempts to distinguish different pathovars and epidemiological types. Subgroups based on such tests are not necessarily hierarchical and their usefulness varies with different diseases.

pv. host
race for cultivars of hos

In contrast to human and mammalian pathogens, the number of genera which include plant pathogens is small. Also, following the introduction of the pathovar concept, the number of species is limited. Most Gram-negative pathogens are in the families Enterobacteriaceae and Pseudomonadaceae. *Agrobacterium tumefaciens* is classed with the symbiotic nitrogen-fixing bacteria, *Rhizobium* spp., in the Rhizobiaceae. The Gram-positive pathogens described here are all coryneform bacteria which, though currently included in the genus *Corynebacterium*, are now being allocated to different genera (see Table 2). None of these pathogens appears closely related to mammallian bacteria though some have affinities with coryneforms from herbage, soil and milk. A *Streptomyces* species which causes potato scab is primarily an opportunistic pathogen and has not been included.

In the Enterobacteriaceae, pathogens diverse in character are grouped together in the genus *Erwinia*. This genus includes pectolytic macergens and necrogens, which have little or no pectolytic activity and cause blight or wilt diseases. Of those pathogens which grow well at 37°C, some are taxonomically closely related to mammalian commensals (mutual feeding without harm) and mammalian pathogens but they have not been implicated in animal disease. The genus also includes a common non-macergenic saprophyte *Erwinia herbicola* (syn. *Enterobacter agglomerans*) which grows at 37°C. (This last species name seems to embrace a diverse group of yellow-pigmented bacteria from both plant an animal sources.) In both plants and animals this organism has occasionally been reported as an opportunistic pathogen.

In the family Pseudomonadaceae, plant pathogens are placed in two genera, *Pseudomonas* and *Xanthomonas*. The first includes both fluorescent and non-fluorescent bacteria and some opportunistic pathogens resembling *P. aeruginosa* and *P. fluorescens*. Most of the truly plant pathogenic *Pseudomonas* spp. are easily distinguishable from saprophytes by two simple diagnostic characters; they are oxidase negative (through lack of cytochrome *c* oxidase) and arginine dihydrolase negative. Such pathogens affect a wide range of plants and are usually highly specific for a particular host. Taxonomically the majority are at present deemed to belong to a single species, *Pseudomonas syringae*, their original species names being used to designate pathovars. Thus the bean pathogen, *P. phaseolicola*, is now referred to as *P. syringae* pv. *phaseolicola* or, for brevity, *P. s. phaseolicola*. No member of this group grows at 37°C and all are distinct from mammalian pathogens. *P. syringae* pathovars are primarily necrogenic but an opportunistic pathogen, which is also oxidase and arginase negative, *P. viridiflava*, is macergenic.

The non-fluorescent *Pseudomonas* spp. are a heterogeneous group and some grow at 37°C. *P. solanacearum*, the most important in economic terms, is closely related to *P. pickettii* which is common in clinical specimens. Others are opportunistic pathogens and include *P. cepacia* which has also been isolated from clinical sources and is related to *P. pseudomallei*, a mammalian pathogen.

Members of the genus *Xanthomonas* affect a wide range of plants. Many are now grouped together as pathovars in the species *X. campestris*. Members of this species produce a unique lipid-soluble yellow pigment; some grow at or near 37°C and appear closely related to *Pseudomonas maltophilia*, a common human commensal. Other *Xanthomonas* spp. form a heterogeneous group; though some are important pathogens (e.g. *X. albilineans*, Table 2), they are not considered further in this book.

Practical work

The study of plant pathogenic bacteria is not difficult. A variety of handbooks give detailed guidance on methods for study of individual pathogens but much can be achieved by beginners with the following:

Plants: beans (germinating seedlings and young plants); tomatoes (young seedlings); potato tubers (whole and sliced).

Pathogens: *P. s. phaseolicola*, *P. s. tomato*, *C. michiganense*, *E. carotovora*, *A. tumefaciens*.

Culture media: yeast-extract peptone agar Ph 6.8–7.2. Sugars or sugar alcohols are often added but development of low pH values can lead to death of stock cultures.

Temperature: 22–30°C (24–27°C is best) for both bacterial cultures and inoculated plants but plants are best kept at lower temperatures at night.

Humidity: high humidity (>99% RH) at night is best (plastic bags can be useful); soil moisture should be high but not excessive.

Beginners can experiment by trying each pathogen on each host plant under different environmental conditions. Methods for preserving cultures are described in various handbooks. Agar-slope cultures must be kept sealed to prevent drying; most will survive well at room temperature.

Terminology

Because this book covers a wide field and will be read by people in different disciplines, simple terminology is important. However, concise and unambiguous definitions of terms are not always possible and the definitions chosen are not necessarily adequate for use outside the context of this book. Readers will need to go to fuller texts for more complete details of the usage of specialized terms.

In plant pathology, terms that have caused most confusion to newcomers are: *hypersensitive reaction* (HR), which is *not* equivalent to the mammalian immune response (Chapter 4) and *virulent* and *avirulent* which are used differently by different pathologists (Chapter 5 and Table 16). The terms *compatible* and *incompatible* (able and unable to coexist) are frequently used though, paradoxically, compatibility in plant-pathogen interactions results in disease. As an aid to further reading, some other terms used in plant pathology are shown in Table 16 of the Glossary.

Further reading

One objective of this book is to provide an introduction to the numerous publications now appearing on this subject. Some guidance is given at the end of each chapter but most major texts, handbooks and practical guides are included in the Bibliography at the end of this book. In the case of multi-author books, the name of the author of a particular chapter may be cited in the text along with the name(s) of the editor(s) of the book listed in the Bibliography; thus: (Cooper in Callow, 1983). Other chapters in these books also provide valuable additional reading.

Other books in this series, *Aspects of Microbiology* (see Bibliography), provide valuable supplementary reading. Where referred to in the text they are cited thus: (Hardy in *Aspects* 4, 1986).

BILLING, E. (1976). The taxonomy of bacteria on the aerial parts of plants. In: *Microbiology of Aerial Plant Surfaces* (edited by C. H. Dickinson and T. F. Preece). Academic Press, London, pp. 223–73.

BOVÉ, J. M. (1984). Wall-less prokaryotes of plants. *Annual Review of Phytopathology* 22: 361–96.

DOWSON, W. J. (1957). *Plant Diseases Due to Bacteria*, 2nd edn. Cambridge University Press, Cambridge.

DYE, D. W., BRADBURY, J. F., GOTO, M., HAYWARD, A. C., LELLIOTT, R. A. and SCHROTH, M. N. (1980). International standards for naming pathovars of phytopathogenic bacteria and a list of pathovar names and pathotype strains. *Review of Plant Pathology* 59: 153–68.

HOLMES, S. (ed.) (1979). *Henderson's Dictionary of Biological Terms*, 9th edn. Longman, London.

SMITH, E. F. (1920). *An Introduction to Bacterial Diseases of Plants*. W. B. Saunders Co., Philadelphia (see also Bibliography).

STAPP, C. (1961). *Bacterial Plant Pathogens*. Oxford University Press, Oxford.

TALBOYS, P. W., GARRETT, C. M. E., AINSWORTH, G. C., PEGG, G. F. and WALLACE, E. R. (1973). *A Guide to the Use of Terms in Plant Pathology*. Commonwealth Mycological Institute, Kew, Surrey.

VIDAVER, A. K. (1982). The plant pathogenic corynebacteria. *Annual Review of Microbiology* 36: 495–517.

2 Host and pathogen

The plant as a habitat

Parallels between mammalian and plant pathogens and their interactions with host tissues and cells are sometimes sought. Though similarities can be found at the cellular level, there are profound differences between the two types of host at the tissue level.

Mammals have circulatory systems (blood and lymph), a sophisticated immune system involving phagocytes (cells which ingest foreign particles), lymphocytes (antibody-forming cells) and complement (a cascading system of enzymes); there are also bactericidal agents such as cationic proteins and iron-binding substances associated with phagocytes and free in the serum. So, the invading bacterium meets a formidal array of lethal agents. In addition there is a memory system whereby responses (antibody formation) on a second encounter are rapid and at a high level and often prevent a second attack of a particular disease. In mammals, in contrast to plants, conditions are frequently anaerobic, the pH is more likely to be alkaline (especially in the intestinal tract) and temperature is regulated over a narrow range (about 37°C in humans) which is outside that for growth of many plant-associated bacteria.

At the cellular level a major difference is that mammalian cells have no walls and cell-cell communication is via surface contact, not via connecting channels as in plants (see Fig. 2). At the enzyme level, lysozyme, which attacks the peptidoglycan of bacterial cell walls, is present in secretions and phagocytes, again equipping mammals well to counter bacterial invaders. Regulatory molecules (hormones) in mammals are often high-molecular-weight glycopeptides with well-defined receptors at sites of action; growth regulators in plants are of low molecular weight and varied composition with ill-defined receptors. Following damage or disease in mammals, healing is a common response, leading to tissue but not organ replacement. In contrast, plants have little capacity for healing. Damaged tissue is usually walled off and, in perennial plants, organs are replaced each season.

The whole plant

Key features of plant anatomy and physiology can be found in standard texts.

Fig. 2 Outline diagrams of transverse (a) and longitudinal (b) sections of a herbaceous dicotyledon stem to show the location of vascular bundles made up of: phloem (nutrient transport), xylem (water transport) and cambium (dividing cells from which xylem and phloem originate). In monocotyledons (such as grains, grasses, onions), the vascular bundles are more scattered. In woody plants, tissue outside the vascular cambium becomes the bark and the xylem becomes a major component of the wood. (c) Diagram of a longitudinal section of stem cortical tissue to show cell components, intercellular spaces and the *symplasm* (continuous space in the plant inside the cytoplasmic membrane) and the *apoplasm* (continuous space outside the cytoplasmic membrane including cell walls and intercellular space).

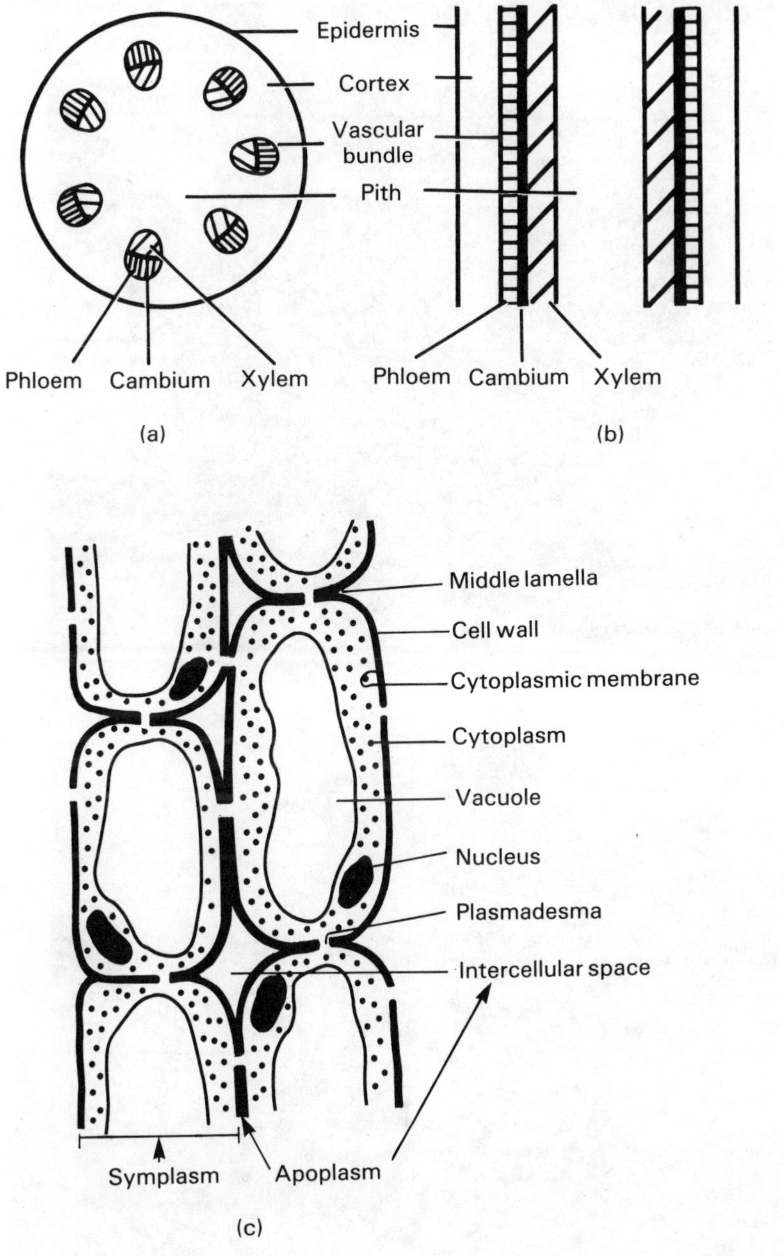
Epidermis
Cortex
Vascular bundle
Pith
Phloem
Cambium
Xylem
(a)
Phloem
Cambium
Xylem
(b)
Middle lamella
Cell wall
Cytoplasmic membrane
Cytoplasm
Vacuole
Nucleus
Plasmadesma
Intercellular space
Symplasm
Apoplasm
(c)

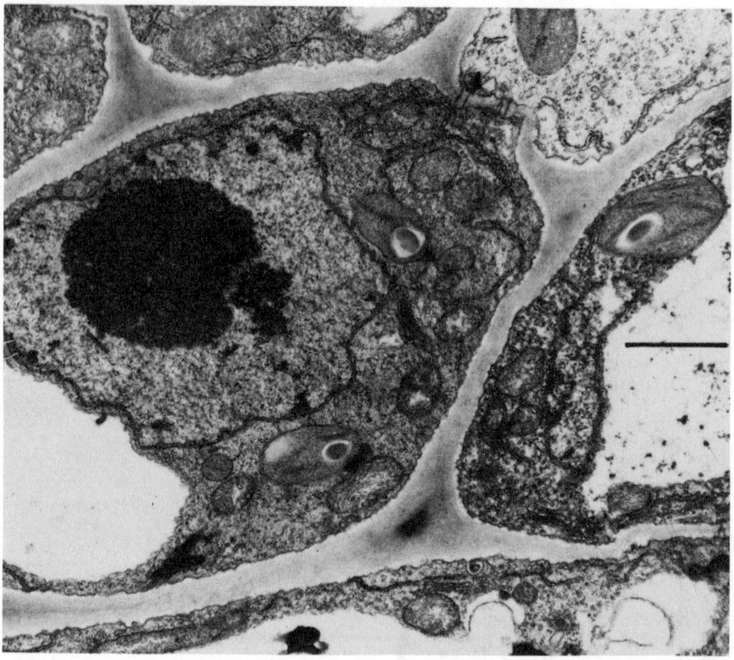

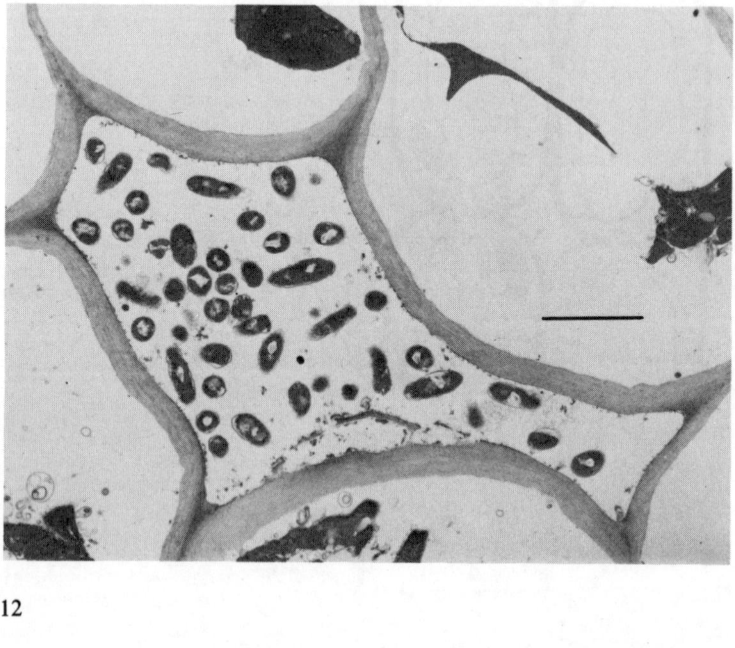

However, since some readers may have little basic knowledge of plant biology, features which are of special importance in bacterial plant diseases are described briefly (see Fig. 2 and Glossary).

Bacterial diseases of plants are largely confined to angiosperms (seeds enclosed in an ovary). Gymnosperms (which include coniferous trees) are not considered, though bacterial involvement in wood rots can be important. Many bacterial pathogens colonize intercellular spaces of parenchyma cells in leaves and stems. Those which invade xylem vessels (vascular pathogens) may also affect adjacent parenchyma cells; functional phloem is only colonized by fastidious prokaryotes.

Although the bulk of water flow from roots to leaves is via xylem vessels, there is significant flow through the *apoplasm*, the continuous intercellular space outside the cytoplasmic membrane (including cell walls, middle lamella and free intercellular space). There is also movement through the *symplasm*, the continuous space inside the cytoplasmic membrane where cells are connected via channels called *plasmadesmata* (Figs. 2 and 3). The concentration of nutrients is very low is xylem vessels and their composition varies in the apoplasm according to diurnal changes and whether or not tissue is importing or exporting nutrients. Water potentials fluctuate widely too. This constant state of flux means that some 'static' experimental systems will not closely resemble normal conditions in plants.

Xylem vessels

Mature xylem vessels are made up of dead, lignified tissue with hydrophobic surfaces. They may vary in length from about 3 cm in an annual plant to as much as 3 m in a tree. Pit membranes on the walls of the vessels allow solutes, but not particles, to move between vessels but the membranes may be degraded during the course of disease. Vertical spread of bacteria in vessels is far more likely than lateral spread. At growing points (root and shoot), where vascular tissue is immature, lateral spread is more easily achieved, both between vessels and from vessels, into parenchymatous tissue. Pressure of bacterial growth and polysaccharide production may aid this process. When a pathogen progresses rapidly up and down a plant it is sometimes assumed to be moving in xylem vessels but with some pathogens movement can also be very rapid in the intercellular spaces of cortical tissue. If a pathogen which normally colonizes cortical tissue enters mature xylem vessels (for example through leaf scars), it is unlikely to travel far or escape, though it may multiply there for long periods without producing external signs of disease.

The levels of nutrients in xylem fluid are very low. The continuous flow of nutrients may suffice initially but not for long. A combination of the bacteria, their polysaccharides, bacteria-induced plant products and air bubbles will block vessels and stop the flow. Vascular pathogens may break down vessel walls and

---

Fig. 3 Transverse sections of healthy and diseased apple stem cortical tissue. (a) Young cells showing membrane-bound organelles, expanding vacuoles and the start of intercellular space formation at angles of cell junctions. Note starch grains in three plastids, also two plasmadesmata (top right wall between two cells). Bar = 15 μm. (b) Large intercellular space between more mature cells, colonized by *Erwinia amylovora*; the surrounding cells have been killed. Bar = 5 μm. (Transmission electron micrographs reproduced by kind permission of the Institute of Horticultural Research, East Malling, Kent (a) and of R.M. Cooper, University of Bath, Avon (b).)

obtain nutrients in this way. Xylem parenchyma cells are another potential source of nutrients if the pathogen induces membrane leakage or death of the plant cells. It is not clear why some pathogens multiply preferentially in xylem vessels rather than in the intercellular spaces of cortical tissue.

This important topic and wilt induction (see Chapter 3) are discussed in detail by van Alfen in Mount and Lacey (1982).

The apoplasm

The composition of primary cells walls varies and most current knowledge comes from study of only a few plant cell types. New methods are now helping to resolve conflicting views on cell wall structure. The simplest concept of the cell wall is that of a moist, cotton mat with pores restricting passage of molecules above a certain size, but this static model has many deficiencies. Bacteria frequently colonize plant tissues where cells are rapidly expanding and laying down new wall material so that, apart from any effects on plant cells induced by the pathogen, there must be constant change at the plant cell wall surface as it matures.

Fibrillar polysaccharides in the walls of parenchymatous tissue of dicotyledons consist mainly of cellulose and the matrix is composed largely of highly branched pectic polymers, a heterogeneous group of polysaccharides, glycoproteins and proteoglycans. The middle lamella contains pectins which are highly esterified; they are slightly branched and serve to cement adjacent cells via calcium and ester cross-links. For possible structures and interconnections see Cooper in Callow (1983). In comparable tissues of some monocotyledons (e.g. grains), there are few if any pectic polymers. The major matrix polysaccharides are either arabinoxylans or β-D-glucans and the cellulose content is low. In other monocotyledons, such as lilies and onions, cell wall composition resembles more closely that of dicotyledons. This is of interest in relation to the host range of *A. tumefaciens* and susceptibility to macergenic *Erwinia* spp.

Proteins in walls of dicotyledons include a strongly basic hydroxyproline-rich glycoprotein (HRGP), which may have a structural role in older cells, as well as enzymes necessary for synthesis and recycling of wall components as the cell expands and matures.

Expanding primary walls of parenchyma cells are thin, plastic and highly hydrated. When cell growth ceases, some walls thicken and in secondary walls there is more xylan and cellulose, less matrix and less water. The amount of HRGP increases and callose deposition, suberization and lignification may occur. The net effect is a structure that is more hydrophobic and more resistant to degradation by bacterial enzymes than the primary cell wall. Pectic enzymes are described in Chapter 3 and changes in cells affecting their resistance to attack in Chapter 4.

In mature plant tissue, the carbon: nitrogen ratio of solutes in the apoplasm may be higher than that in young tissue. In both types of tissue there is diurnal variation. The pH at cell wall surfaces varies but tends to be acidic rather than alkaline. Oxygen levels are normally high unless tissue remains water-soaked. Much uncertainty remains about the precise nature and properties of the cell wall surfaces that are colonized by pathogens. For details of current concepts concerning cell walls see Roberts *et al.* (1985).

Pectic polymers

Of all cell wall constituents, pectic polymers are the most readily degraded by bacteria (both saprophytes and pathogens). On restricted hydrolysis, various polymers can be distinguished. The backbone of the main polymer is rhamnogalacturan, which is made up of long chains of α-1, 4-linked galacturonic acid (*Gal A*) (see Fig. 5) interspersed with 1, 2-linked L-rhamnose units. Linked to the backbone are galactan and araban side-chains. The *Gal A* carboxyl groups are methylated to varying degrees; the general term *pectin* applies to such polymers. High-methoxyl pectins are soluble in water and form viscous solutions; low-methoxyl pectins are less soluble. Non-esterified carboxyl groups may be cross-linked by calcium or magnesium to form bridges between chains and insoluble gels form which have ion-exchange properties with some selectivity for calcium and heavy-metal ions. During fruit ripening such gels are converted to soluble pectic polymers so that the tissue softens. Tissue maceration involves breakdown of pectic substances in the middle lamella and the cell wall so that cells separate and cell membrane integrity is lost. The action of pectic enzymes is described in Chapter 3.

Cytoplasmic membranes and membrane-bound organelles

Membranes are easily perturbed and the manner of this perturbation by plant pathogens is a major area of study. Less is known about membranes in plants than in mammals and bacteria because the plant cell wall interferes with their study; but the basic structure is thought to be similar in all these organisms. With plant, as with bacterial membranes, glycolipids are common. Like glycoproteins, glycolipids might be involved in signal/receptor systems. The nature of specific receptors has proved elusive in plants.

There are some major differences between plant and mammalian cell organelles, including plastids. Some plastids (chloroplasts) are concerned with photosynthesis; others contain carotenoid pigments or store starch. The fire blight pathogen is called *E. amylovora* (starch consuming) because starch (amylose) grains disappear during the course of the disease, not because it has the ability to hydrolyze starch. In addition, mature plant cells have a large membrane-bound vacuole which plays a major role in regulating cell water content and maintaining cell turgor; damage to this membrane (the tonoplast) means rapid cell death. The vacuole is also a reservoir for hydrolytic enzymes and for a variety of organic molecules, including phenolic substances, sugars and glycosides, which on release are readily hydrolyzed by plant enzymes. Products of hydrolysis include highly toxic hydrogen cyanide (HCN), in cyanogenic plants, and phenolics which may be converted to toxic quinones. Apart from any effect on bacterial growth, polyphenols inhibit the activity of pectic and other enzymes. Thus, death of the plant cell is a perilous event for the invading pathogen unless it has the means either to detoxify these substances, tolerate their presence or escape beyond their influence. HCN detoxifying systems (found in some fungi) have not so far been demonstrated in plant pathogenic bacteria attacking cyanogenic plants. Nor do toxic phenolic compounds appear to present a major problem. Rotting plant tissue is soon colonized by a wide variety of saprophytic aerobic and anaerobic bacteria.

Nevertheless, pathogenic bacteria survive best at the leading edges of infected plant tissue. Attempts to isolate pathogens from dead tissue often fail and, in disease diagnosis, the junction between dead and living tissues is the recommended point for making isolations. The precise role in disease resistance of preformed antimicrobial substances and their products is still largely a matter for conjecture

(Schobeck and Grunewaldt-Stocker in Gould *et al.*, 1986). Other consequences of plant cell death are discussed in Chapter 4.

Nutrient availability

There is little definitive information on transport of nutrients to sites of infection for bacterial plant diseases but certain assumptions seem reasonable from available observations. Bacteria multiplying in intercellular spaces (Fig. 3) need to intercept nutrients which diffuse through the apoplasm via hydrated cell walls. It is important to know whether the apoplasm can supply adequate nutrients and water for initial multiplication and how the pathogen acquires further nutrients and water to reach population levels sufficient to produce lesions in plant tissue.

Using data from published observations, Hancock and Huisman (1981) calculated that in the case of *P. s. phaseolicola* there was probably sufficient nutrients in the walls of a single cell to support 60 bacteria and that, with diffusion from the apoplast of nearby non-infected leaf areas, 10^7 bacteria per cm^2 of leaf could be supported. Other research workers have reached similar conclusions. Thus, it may only need mild leakage from host plant cells in the affected area to support bacterial populations normally observed in infected leaves and it is unnecessary to consider long-distance transport of nutrients to the site of infection. However, leaf lesions normally remain restricted; the same arguments may not apply to other tissues where rapid bacterial cell multiplication and disease progression is necessary.

Water relationships

As in other branches of microbiology, this is a recurring theme. Unfortunately, water relationships are sometimes ignored because of difficulties of measurement and of standardization in experimental systems. Different terms are used to describe water potential values in different disciplines. As a broad guide, a comparison of values at 20°C is given in Table 3; these values are not applicable at other temperatures.

The bacterial pathogen needs to obtain water for growth and, at times, to move in a water film. For optimal growth, water potential (ψ) values above -5 bar are usually necessary whereas fungi may show optimal growth between -5 and -15 bar. For movement in tissue by means of flagella, soil studies suggest that values above -1 bar would be necessary to provide a water film on cell wall surfaces. During daylight, when transpiration rates are high, ψ in the leaf may often fall below -20 bar; at night it may approach zero, depending on the soil moisture. Where this and soil temperature and air humidity are high, ψ may reach positive values and guttation droplets may be seen at leaf margins where there are hydathodes; such conditions can favour entry of bacteria into leaf tissue (see Chapter 4). In stem cortical tissue, ψ will fluctuate less widely.

Low ψ values have other effects on bacteria. They can cause a prolonged lag in growth and affect the efficiency of substrate utilization and of enzyme activity, including pectic. The general rule is that bacterial diseases are initiated and progress at high rates when ψ is near zero and temperatures are near optimal but they are seriously restricted in dry conditions. There may, however, be sudden collapse of diseased plant tissue in hot dry weather because the plant can no longer tolerate

Table 3 Relationships of osmotic potential, water potential, relative humidity and water activity to sucrose molality and molal- and molar-based sucrose solutions (*approximate* equivalents at 20°C)

		Sucrose		
π or ψ[a] (bars)	% RH ($a_w \times 10^2$)	Molality (m)	Molal soln (m) mol $kg^{-1} \times 10^{-1}$)	Molar soln (M) mol $dm^{-3} \times 10^{-1}$ (%w/v)
0	100.00	0.00	0.00	0.00
−1	99.93	0.04	1.40	1.38
−5	99.63	0.20	6.86	6.57
−10	99.26	0.39	13.51	12.45
−15[b]	98.90	0.58	19.85	17.65
−20	98.53	0.76	26.01	22.31
−25	98.17	0.93	31.97	26.65
−30	97.80	1.10	37.71	30.52

[a] π, osmotic potential; ψ, water potential; RH, relative humidity; a_w, water activity.
[b] Bacterial growth rates are markedly reduced at values below this point.
(Data from various sources. For detailed data see Parr *et al.*, 1981)

the water stress. This can give the false impression that dry conditions favour disease.

The bacterium as a pathogen

The cell

All plant pathogenic bacteria are rod-shaped. Spore-forming *Bacillus* and *Clostridium* species are only associated with storage rots, not with field diseases. Gram-positive pathogens are confined to the coryneform bacteria which, unlike many Gram-positive bacteria, lack teichoic acids in their cell walls.

The necrogenic and macergenic *Erwinia* species belong to the family Enterobacteriaceae so, in some but not all respects, *Escherichia coli* and related bacteria may be good models. When considering interactions between plant and bacterial cell surfaces it is worth bearing in mind the zones of adhesion demonstrated in the cell envelope of *E. coli*. These correspond to sites of export of extracellular polysaccharides (EPS) and lipopolysaccharides (LPS), of insertion of outer membrane proteins, of adsorption for some bacteriocins and bacteriophages and of uptake of siderophores (iron chelators) and various metabolites. Plant pathogenic pseudomonads differ in many respects from *P. aeruginosa* so it is difficult to judge how far this organism can serve as a model. EPS and LPS production by plant pathogenic bacteria is described in Chapter 3.

Descriptions of the difference between Gram-positive and Gram-negative bacteria can be found elsewhere (see for example Priest in *Aspects of Microbiology* 9, 1984; Rogers in *Aspects* 6, 1983) but a few points are worth emphasis. Gram-positive bacteria have a thick peptidoglycan layer outside the cytoplasmic membrane and hydrolytic enzymes are commonly liberated into the surrounding medium. In Gram-negative bacteria, the peptidoglycan forms a thin layer over the cytoplasmic membrane and beyond this there is a lipid-rich outer membrane. Between the two membranes lies the periplasm which contains amino acid and sugar-binding proteins and hydrolytic enzymes. Some enzymes are extracellular and are released into the surrounding medium. Such enzymes include pectic and other cell wall degrading enzymes of importance in pathogenicity (see Chapter 3). Current knowledge concerning non-pathogenic Gram-positive bacteria is not necessarily applicable to plant pathogenic coryneforms, because the latter have not been studied in detail but they are likely to differ from Gram-negative pathogens in their susceptibility to antibacterial agents.

With the exception of some coryneforms, most plant pathogens are motile. The flagella of plant pathogens are polar (*Pseudomonas*, *Xanthomonas*) or peritrichous (*Erwinia*, *Agrobacterium*) and are important for chemotaxis and entry into plant tissue. Fimbriae (pili) in plant pathogens have not been extensively studied; they have been attributed a role in adhesion to plant surfaces but not so far in the specific fashion observed with mammalian pathogens. EPS, as with mammalian pathogens, appears to have a major role in pathogenicity at least in the case of necrogens; the role of LPS is less certain (see Chapter 3).

Some bacteria produce yellow lipid-soluble pigments, notably *X. campestris* pvs and the Gram-positive coryneforms; occasionally, other water-insoluble pigments are seen. Most *P. syringae* pvs produce water-soluble fluorescent green pigments which chelate iron. Pink, water-soluble pigments are produced by *E. rhapontici* and *P. pastinaceae*.

Physiology

Nutrition Various special media have been recommended for the isolation of different plant pathogens but many grow and survive well on a yeast extract-peptone medium at pH 6.8–7.2. Growth may be improved by adding sugars or sugar alcohols but there is a danger that cultures will die rapidly if the pH falls greatly and there may be excessive slime formation. Many plant pathogens will grow on a simple defined medium with an inorganic source of nitrogen but some require one or more growth factors, most commonly nicotinic acid, thiamine or biotin. Some xanthomonads and most coryneform pathogens require amino acids, in particular sulphur-containing ones such as l-methionine.

Ease of growth and survival on laboratory media does not mean that these pathogens can grow saprophytically and survive under field conditions in the absence of a specific host plant. Most fail to persist in the field, i.e. they are obligate parasites. *P. syringae* pvs can only use a narrow range of carbon-energy sources compared with the saprophyte *P. fluorescens*. This suggests that through evolution in association with plants *P. syringae* pvs are now less well adapted to a saprophytic existence. Of the *P. syringae* pvs, only *P. s. pisi* can utilize homoserine; this is a dominant amino acid in pea plants and suggests adaptation to a particular host plant.

Temperature Plant pathogens vary in their optimal temperature for growth but for most it lies between 25 and 30°C. Many show diminished growth above 30°C (*E. amylovora*, *P. syringae* pvs) but some still grow well up to about 35°C (*X. campestris* pvs *P. solanacearum*). *P. syringae* pvs and other pathogens multiply at 0°C but only very slowly. These temperature requirements have sometimes proved a problem in taxonomic studies; also, rapid diagnostic techniques often require high temperatures of incubation. There are practical problems in laboratories where it is difficult to maintain an incubator at 25°C without artificial cooling.

Under field conditions the pathogen must contend with temperatures that can fluctuate widely between day and night and from day to day. However, a plant pathogen held at a low temperature can respond very rapidly to a rise in temperature. Water relationships need to be considered alongside temperature relationships because each affects the other. The growth of the plant is also affected by temperature and water availability and this in turn affects the environment for bacterial growth. The successful pathogen must be adapted to exploit all the subtle changes that occur.

The temperature requirements of a pathogen often reflect the climatic area where the disease it causes is most severe. Among the macergens, *E. chrysanthemi* is more important in sub-tropical areas and on glasshouse crops whilst *E. c. atroseptica* is largely confined to potato crops in temperate climates; *E. c. carotovora* is intermediate. *P. syringae* pvs are more commonly a problem in cooler climates or during cooler periods of the growing season. *X. c. campestris* pvs are favoured by warm weather and the same is largely true for *P. solanacearum*. *E. amylovora* causes little disease at temperatures below 18°C (though it still grows and infections will progress) but disease spread and progression within tissue largely ceases when temperatures exceed 30°C.

Oxygen Most plant pathogens are strictly aerobic. The exceptions are *Erwinia* species but of these only the macergens grow well in culture media under anaerobic conditions. *E. amylovora* grows poorly and so does the common epiphyte *E. herbicola*. Unlike the saprophyte *P. fluorescens*, *P. syringae* pvs do not produce arginine dihydrolase and cannot grow anaerobically in the presence of arginine. Nor can they grow anaerobically in the presence of nitrate, as can some denitrifying strains of *P. fluorescens*. Also, unlike *P. fluorescens*, they lack cytochrome *c* oxidase and fail to produce H_20_2. It seems that cytochrome *c* oxidase is most commonly associated with bacteria growing in a nutritionally poor environment where they must conserve energy (Elstner, 1982). This may be an example of a mutation which has parasitic advantages. It could mean that such pathogens are at less risk from the oxidation of phenolic substances released from damaged tissue (Moustafa and Whittenbury, 1970). Differences in the respiratory systems of pathogens have also been suggested as a factor in their much greater sensitivity, compared with *P. fluorescens*, to optical brighteners such as cationic benzoxazole compounds (Gonzalez-Lopez *et al.* 1981).

Siderophores These have been detected in plant pathogens and some plant-associated bacteria produce water-soluble pigments which chelate iron. So far, there is little evidence that siderophores could be important in pathogenicity but work in this area is still at an early stage. It remains to be seen whether plants are as well equipped as mammals to frustrate invading bacteria by binding iron or other essential metals.

Extracellular enzymes Both Gram-positive and Gram-negative pathogens produce a variety of extracellular hydrolytic enzymen. Some *X. campestris* pvs produce amylase but most of the enzymes secreted which are associated with plant cell wall or membrane degradation are cellulases, xylanases, pectinases, proteinases and (more rarely) phospholipases. Only the pectic enzymes have been extensively studied (see Chapter 3). Opportunistic and wide host-range pathogens are among the most active producers of hydrolytic enzymes. It is sometimes difficult to judge the importance of enzymes in particular pathogens because tests *in vitro* may poorly reflect production and activity *in vivo*.

Serology

As in other fields of study, serological techniques have proved powerful tools in plant bacteriology and methods used differ little from those used elsewhere. Like phage-sensitivity tests they can (but often fail to) show the desired degree of specificity, for example at the pathovar level. The significance of seemingly specific antigens in relation to host specificity is not clear. Antigens shared between host and pathogen have been sought but not often found. Monoclonal antibodies should make identification using serological methods more precise. The value of serological methods in the study of plant pathogens and future prospects are discussed by Halk and De Boer (1985). Slade and Tiffin (1984) give an account of serological studies on macergenic, necrogenic and saprophytic *Erwinia* spp.

Phages and bacteriocins

The phages lysing plant pathogenic bacteria vary widely in character but are comparable to those lysing other bacteria. They have been used in diagnosis and in epidemiological studies and for selection of avirulent mutants of pathogens (Billing and Garrett, 1980; Persley, in Fahy and Persley, 1983). They can be isolated from a wide variety of sources including sewage, manure, rotting meat, soil and healthy and infected plants, especially when the disease is well developed. Sometimes, but not invariably, the infected plants are the best source of phages showing a high degree of specificity. Specificity at the pathovar level is often elusive, especially in *X. campestris*.

The bacteriocins of plant pathogenic bacteria have received little attention, except as potential disease control agents. In plant pathology the term has not been confined to proteins and clear distinction is not often made between high- and low-molecular-weight products, though the latter are sometimes referred to as antibiotics. The agent used for control of crown gall, Agrocin 84, is a low-molecular-weight nucleotide.

It is tempting to think that some lessons learned from bacterium-bacteriocin interactions might be applicable to interactions between necrogenic bacteria and plant cells. Some bacteriocins kill by increasing membrane permeability, others penetrate membranes and act intracellularly as DNases or RNases. All bacteriocins bind to receptors on the outer cell membrane; some are transported via channels associated with uptake of iron-chelating agents, nucleosides or other molecules. Many bacteriocins, like phages, show a high degree of host specificity.

Fungal plant pathogens

Some differences between fungal and bacterial pathogens are worth emphasis. Fungi are eukaryotes and have complex morphological features and life cycles. Spread of disease is commonly by spore dispersal. Some fungi can penetrate plant surfaces and tissue invasion (via intercellular spaces or in xylem vessels) involves hyphal growth and sometimes specialized structures. Fungi have chitin and/or glucans, not peptidoglycan, in their cell walls and some have sterols in their membranes. Most grow well at low pH levels and are more tolerant than bacteria of low water potentials.

Many fungi fall into two main groups on the basis of nutritional strategy: *biotrophs*, which depend on living host cells and may penetrate cell walls, must ensure that cell death is delayed; *necrotrophs* feed off dead cells and so require rapid host cell death. Other fungi, *hemibiotrophs*, appear to have a short biotrophic phase followed by a necrotrophic phase. Many, but not all, necrotrophs produce cell wall degrading enzymes and have a relatively wide host range. Biotrophs cause minimal host cell wall breakdown and have a narrow host range; they are often difficult or impossible to grow in culture. Macergenic bacteria have much in common with necrotrophic fungi. Some researchers consider necrogenic and oncogenic bacteria to be biotrophic or hemibiotrophic but they are very different from many fungal biotrophs.

In spite of the many differences between fungal and bacterial plant pathogens some of their basic strategies in plant pathogenicity are very similar. In bacteria, EPS production seems to be of greater importance in pathogenicity but the role of extracellular fungal polysaccharides is largely unknown. For direct comparisons see Goodman *et al.* (1986) and for further information on fungal pathogens see Agrios (1978), Callow (1982) and Dickinson and Lucas (1982).

Further reading

BILLING, E. and GARRETT, C. M. E. (1980). *Phages in the Identification of Plant Pathogenic Bacteria* (edited by M. Goodfellow and R. G. Board). Academic Press, London, pp. 319–38.

CALLOW, J. A. (1982). Molecular aspects of fungal infection. In: *The Molecular Biology of Plant Development* (edited by H. Smith and D. Grierson). Blackwell Scientific Publications, Oxford, pp. 467–97.

DICKINSON, C. H. and LUCAS, J. A. (1982). *Plant Pathology and Plant Pathogens*, 2nd edition. Blackwell Scientific Publications, Oxford.

GONZALEZ-LOPEZ, J., RHODES-ROBERTS, M. E., PATON, A. M. and FENLON, D. (1981). The selective activity of a benzoxazole brightener against phytopathogenic bacteria. *Journal of Applied Bacteriology* 50: 319–34.

HALK, E. L. and DE BOER, S. H. (1985). Monoclonal antibodies in plant disease research. *Annual Review of Phytopathology* 23: 321–50.

HANCOCK, J. G. and HUISMAN, O. C. (1981). Nutrient movement in host-pathogen systems. *Annual Review of Phytopathology* 19: 309–31.

MOUSTAFA, F. A. and WHITTENBURY, R. (1970). Properties which appear to allow phytopathogenic pseudomonads to counteract plant defence mechanisms. *Phytopathologische Zeitschrift* 67: 214–24.

PARR, J. F., GARDNER, W. R. and ELIOTT, L. F. (eds) (1981). *Water Potential Relations in Soil Microbiology*, SSSA Special Publication No. 9. Soil Science Society of America, Madison, Wisconsin.

SLADE, M. B. and TIFFIN, A. I. (1984). Biochemical and serological characterization of *Erwinia*. In: *Methods in Microbiology*, Vol. 15 (edited by T. Bergen). Academic Press, London, pp. 227–93.

SLATYER, R. O. (1967). *Plant-Water Relationships*. Academic Press, London.

3 Pathogenicity and virulence factors

For maximum pathogenic potential it is important for invading bacteria to colonize tissue rapidly and to reach high population levels before plant tissue maturation or other plant responses limit bacterial growth. In turn, for plant resistance to be most effective, resistance mechanisms must be capable of rapid and massive mobilization. Plant responses are discussed in Chapter 4, whereas in this chapter some of the weapons in the armoury of the pathogen are considered. In addition to producing specific virulence factors, successful pathogens are sometimes able to increase the susceptibility of the host; they must also avoid provoking plant resistance reactions.

Ideally, pathogen products with a major role in *pathogenicity* (ability to produce disease) should be distinguished from those affecting *virulence* (ability to increase disease severity) but this is not always easy. In mammalian diseases (see Brubaker, 1985) many pathogenicity and virulence factors may be produced by the pathogen to counter the immune system, to prevent phagocytosis and to avoid being killed following phagocyte ingestion or by antibacterial agents in serum. Plant pathogens invading tissue do not need to attach to specific sites, as do some mammalian pathogens on mucous membrane surfaces, to avoid being dislodged from an ideal position; in fact, in plants, attachment could be a disadvantage and limit disease progression. Most high-molecular-weight toxins produced by mammalian pathogens (Stephen and Pietrowski in *Aspects* 2, 1986) would seem to have little direct relevance to toxins produced by plant pathogens. Indirectly, however, something might be learned from their mode of action at the cellular level, especially in the case of toxins inducing leakage of cell electrolytes.

Polysaccharides

These may occur in the form of rigid or deformable capsules on the bacteria or as free, water-soluble or insoluble polymers; Both forms may be present together. Their presence in microscopic preparations may not be obvious unless special stains are used; ruthenium red, useful in electron microscopy, also stains pectic substances so care is needed in interpretating observations. Similarly, with light microscopy, dry stained films can produce artifacts. Wet India ink preparations are more reliable, provided the capsule is sufficiently rigid to prevent penetration of ink particles.

Much has been written about surface polysaccharides in relation to microbial ecology and mammalian pathology. An outline of the range of roles attributed to these polysaccharides follows. The bacterial capsule has been described as: a thick, continuous, highly ordered, hydrated, non-toxic gel which is usually polyanionic; a network with pores and channels; a molecular sieve; and an ion-exchange resin. It gives the bacterium a hydrophilic surface and a means of modifying the microenvironment in a variety of ways. It extends the area of surface for cell activity but rapid diffusion is prevented (an unstirred layer). The capsule will affect access of ions (including protons), attract and concentrate nutrients and hold extracellular enzymes. It will also absorb and bind water, thus buffering the bacterial cell against rapid hydration and dehydration and promoting survival.

Apart from facilitating rapid bacterial multiplication, capsules and EPS can protect against inhibitory agents, including polycationic peptides, surface-active agents, heavy-metal ions (by binding or chelation), antibiotics, phages and bacteriocins and (in mammalian disease) antibodies and phagocytosis. The presence of such inhibitory agents may sometimes select mutants from a bacterial population which are more heavily capsulated and so better able to survive. On surfaces, EPS may help to overcome electrostatic forces, thus aiding initial binding and, later, helping to make adhesion firmer (see Marsh and Martin in *Aspects* 1, 1984). In contrast, in some mammalian diseases, EPS-producing pathogens prove more invasive; this is thought to be related to the composition of the EPS. The same could be true in plant disease.

Conditions favouring production of EPS may differ with individual organisms and it is difficult to generalize. The following have been found favourable in individual cases: media containing a high carbon:nitrogen ratio; low levels of nitrogen, phosphorous, sulphur or potassium; good aeration; a solid surface; temperatures suboptimal for growth. The effect on host physiology must also be considered. Environmental factors may affect chemical composition, conformation and molecular size which can itself be variable under a single set of conditions. This is considered further in relation to wilt induction later in this chapter.

Before considering in detail the role of EPS in plant pathogenesis, the different types which may be produced by the same bacterium should be distinguished. The *homopolysaccharide* levan (a polyfructosan) is commonly produced by necrogenic plant pathogens, including *P. syringae* pvs and *E. amylovora*, and by a variety of saprophytic bacteria, especially *P. fluorescens*. It is produced extracellularly in the presence of sucrose and related sugars and is the dominant polysaccharide when such bacteria are grown on media containing 5% (w/v) sucrose. Levan-producing bacterial colonies are usually large, domed and show a radial structure. Like *dextran* (a polyglucosan), levan does not require sugar nucleotides or lipid intermediates for its synthesis. It is commonly insoluble in water but not associated with capsulation. The role, if any, of levan in pathogenicity or virulence and the extent to which it is produced in infected plants is not known.

The discussion which follows is concerned with extracellular *heteropolysaccharides* produced by plant pathogens. A variant strain which fails to produce adequate EPS *in vivo* at an early stage is likely to be at a grave disadvantage compared with the fully competent wild-type. Such variants can be isolated from diseased plants and from laboratory cultures indicating that both genotypic and phenotypic variation in bacterial populations, *in vivo* and *in vitro*, is possible (see Chapter 5).

Many polysaccharides contain acyl groups, *0*-acetyl, pyruvate and ketal groups being the most common. Any specificity residing in the EPS molecule is likely to be influenced by such groups (Sutherland, 1985) and they deserve further study in plant pathogenic bacteria. Thus, although all *X. campestris* pvs seem to produce a similar EPS, xanthan, and *P. syringae* pvs perhaps commonly produce alginates, differences in the level and type of acylation might be key determinants of specificity. In *E. amylovora* and *E. herbicola*, acylation may explain minor antigenic

Table 4 Extracellular polysaccharides[a]

Characteristics	*E. amylovora*	*X. campestris* pvs	*P. syringae* pvs	*P. solanacearum*
Trivial name	Amylovorin	Xanthan	Alginate	
Acidity	Acid	Acid	Acid	Neutral
Glucose	+	+		+
Galactose	+			
Mannose	+	+		
Rhamnose				+
Galactosamine				+
Glucuronic acid	+	+		
Mannuronic acid			+	
Guluronic acid			+	
Acetate		+	+	+
Pyruvate	+	+		
Succinate	+			

[a] Data from various sources; sometimes provisional. In EPS from coryneform pathogens the following components have been reported: glucose, galactose, fucose, mannose, rhamnose, aldobiuronic acid.

differences in their polysaccharides which otherwise appear identical (see Slade and Tiffin, 1984).

Some components of EPS from different pathogens are shown in Table 4. In some of the cases shown, detailed structures including linkages and side chains have been determined. LPS side-chains show different components; rhamnose is common in *Pseudomonas* LPS and fucose is present in LPS from *E. amylovora*. Glucose, galactose and hexosamines have been found in LPS from other pathogens. At present no characteristics of core or side-chain LPS clearly distinguish plant pathogens from other Gram-negative bacteria.

Roles of polysaccharides in plant pathogenicity

Many roles for EPS can be envisaged from the list of properties described, ranging from survival outside the host and within plant tissue to chelation of metals, nutrient uptake and water retention. Water retention has received most attention and related to this are possible roles in suppression of the hypersensitive reaction, HR (see Chapter 4).

Since water retention in intercellular spaces is of primary importance for the growth of pathogenic bacteria, EPS production has obvious advantages. Indeed, a variety of bacteria will grow in intercellular spaces and HR induction is prevented if tissue is kept water-soaked (for example by keeping plants under high humidity after infiltration with water or agar). Persistent water soaking of tissue is a characteristic early symptom in diseases caused by many necrogenic pathogens and there is no doubt that EPS has a role here.

Infiltration of EPS into leaves, though not inducing plant cell leakage, can lead to persistent water soaking of the infiltrated area if plants are kept under high relative humidity (El-Banoby and Rudolph, 1979). EPS from a particular pathogen seems to be more effective in maintaining water soaking in a compatible host or cultivar than in an incompatible one but these findings need substantiation in other systems. Other work suggests that infiltration with EPS of different types (levan, alginate, xanthan) from plant pathogenic bacteria may enhance multiplication rates of bacteria in leaf tissue but the response seems to vary according to experimental conditions.

Study of xanthan, the EPS produced by *X. campestris* pvs has suggested that conformation of the polysaccharide may be important in pathogenicity (Morris *et al.*, 1977). Xanthan interacts with other polysaccharides which have a β-1, 4-linked backbone, such as cellulose, forming a gel. This does not account for host specificity but it might indicate adaptation of the pathogen to the plant environment. Stable gels are probably important for water retention but whether a specific interaction between pathogen and host polysaccharides is necessary needs further investigation.

The physical properties of EPS may be important in many respects. The EPS produced by *E. amylovora* (Fig. 4) can vary at low humidities from a hard brittle texture to a soft gum which can be pulled out into fine strands easily blown in the wind. At high humidities it becomes sticky and readily adheres to insects or pruning tools. All these forms are rapidly dispersed by water. Xanthan has wide and diverse commercial applications, including use as a stabilizer, an emulsifier, a thickener and a lubricant.

It has long been thought that LPS might be important in host specificity and in HR induction. There is little direct evidence for this but any alteration in LPS composition usually results in reduced virulence or in avirulence. Considering the important role of endotoxin in mammalian disease, and the lipid-A component in particular, it would be surprising if LPS had no role in plant disease, unless

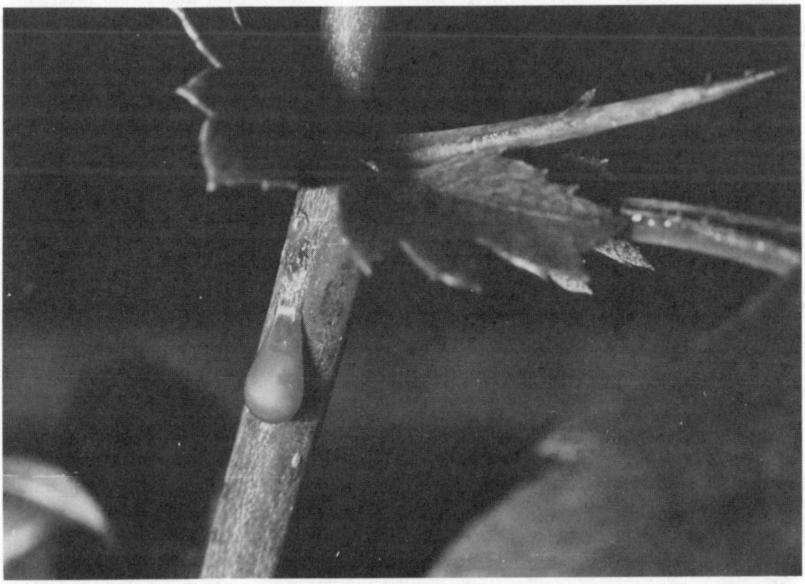

Fig. 4 Bacterial ooze (*E. amylovora*) on hawthorn (X5). The pathogen is surrounded by bacterial polysaccharide; sorbitol from the plant is also present. (Reproduced by kind permission of The Institute of Horticultural Research, East Malling, Kent.)

endotoxin activity depends largely on physiological and immune system factors not found in plants.

Wilt induction by EPS

Major vascular wilt pathogens include *C. m. insidiosum*, *C. m. michiganense*, *C. m. sepedonicum*, *C. flaccumfaciens*, *E. stewartii*, *E. chrysanthemi*, *P. solanacearum*, *X. c. campestris* and *X. c. oryzae*. All colonize xylem vessels and produce EPS. With many other EPS-producing pathogens which primarily colonize cortical tissue, wilt is associated with necrotic lesions. However, with the vascular wilt pathogens, extensive wilt may be seen well beyond the sites of colonization and is not associated with necrosis. This is described in detail by Van Alfen in Mount and Lacey (1982) and only an outline of some of the factors concerned follows here.

Simple colonization of a proportion of plant xylem vessels does not account for the extensive wilt which may follow. Cell wall degrading enzymes (CWDE) and other agents, including ethylene produced by the bacteria or the host plant, contribute to symptoms of bacterial wilt caused by *P. solanacearum*. Extensive cell wall degradation in bacterial wilt of tomato (*C. m. michiganense*) suggests that CWDE have a major role in this disease. In these and other wilt diseases, EPS may still be important in the restriction of water movement. EPS can be active at very low levels but as the mode of action is physical rather than chemical it can be confusing to refer to EPS as a toxin.

To cause extensive restriction of water flow, EPS must pass out of the colonized vessels (already non-functional) to functional vessels; it may also accumulate on pit membranes and at petiole junctions where pore sizes are too small to allow further passage. EPS molecules may vary in size and in a disease such as alfalfa wilt (*C. m. insidiosum*), some may pass on and accumulate in primary cell walls of leaves to produce wilt of leaf tissue. Whilst some degree of host specificity may lie in the EPS produced by a particular pathogen, other polysaccharides are often equally effective in producing wilt symptoms in experimental systems such as the cut shoot test. The EPS may have another function in invaded vessels—contributing to a build up of pressure which aids movement of the bacteria there. Where there is no other escape, the combined pressure of bacterial growth and its surrounding polysaccharide matrix may sometimes split weaker vessels. In woody plants this may produce blisters under the bark which break when the bark becomes wet.

Pectic enzymes

The complexity of the subject of pectic enzymes is reflected in the terminology used, including alternative names and abbreviations and qualifications concerning the activity of different enzymes. Table 5 and Fig. 5 are provided for guidance but the reality is more complex. For further information see Chatterjee and Vidaver (1986), Chesson (1980), and Cooper in Callow (1983).

There is a variety of pectic enzymes. *endo*-enzymes produce random cleavage and cause a rapid decrease in viscosity of pectin solutions. *Exo*-enzymes produce terminal cleavage and a slow decrease in viscosity. Tissue maceration is largely a result of pectic *endo*-enzyme activity but proteolytic enzymes may also play a part.

Table 5 Major pectic enzymes produced by bacteria and fungi

Enzyme type	Abbreviations	Optimum pH	Produced mainly by
Hydrolase			
endo-polygalacturonase	*endo*-PG	4–5	Fungi[a]
Lyase (transeliminase)			
endo-polygalacturonide (pectic) lyase	*endo*-PL or PGL	8–10[b]	Bacteria
endo-polymethyl galacturonide (pectin) lyase	*endo*-PL or PML	8–10[b]	Fungi
Methylesterase (pectin esterase)			
pectin methylesterase	PE or PME	7–9 4–6	Bacteria Fungi

[a] Produced by plants during fruit ripening.
[b] Ca^{2+} requirement.
[c] Present in walls of healthy plants.

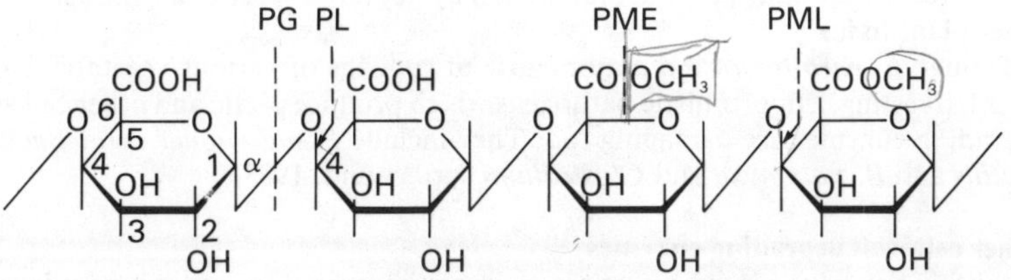

Fig. 5 Sites of action of pectic enzymes. PG, polygalacturonase; PL, pectic lyase; PML, pectin lyase; PME, pectin methylesterase.

There are two classes of pectic *endo*-enzymes, hydrolases and lyases (trans-eliminases which cause β-elimination). Some enzymes are sensitive to the degree of methylation of the rhamnogalacturanan; a further enzyme type, pectin methylesterase (PME), can have a role but little is known about PME production by plant pathogenic bacteria. The lyases have a high optimal pH for activity and require calcium. In the macerating *Erwinia* spp., *endo*-polygalacturonide (pectic) lyase (PL, PGL) is the most important enzyme, though others may be involved. Multiple forms (isozymes) of both the hydrolase *endo*-polygalacturonase (PG) and PL have been described which differ in optimal requirements for activity. Their significance is uncertain but they could increase the versatility of the pathogen.

PL synthesis by macergenic *Erwinia* spp., which are facultative anaerobes, is stimulated by anaerobiosis and it is possible that the rate and quantity of enzyme excreted by these pathogens under anerobic conditions is one factor that distinguishes them from saprophytic pectolytic bacteria.

A sequel to plant tissue maceration is cell death with release of water and of utilizable carbon-energy and nitrogen sources for nutrition of the pathogen. But there are many other consequences of cell death, some of which are unfavourable either for the pathogen or for pectic enzyme synthesis or both.

The simplest explanation for plant cell death caused by pectic enzymes is that cell wall damage leads to osmotic fragility and loss of cell turgor. However, changes in plant cells, including leakage of ions, may occur before obvious signs of cell wall damage suggesting that there may be other preceding or aggravating factors. In macergenic *Erwinia* spp. there seems little doubt that pectic enzyme production and export is essential for pathogenicity.

So far, attempts to demonstrate pectic enzyme activity *in vitro* or *in vivo* in *E. amylovora* have failed. Pectic enzyme production by *P. syringae* and *X. campestris* pvs and coryneform pathogens has not been extensively studied. There is some uncertainty whether these pathogens produce PL or PG or both; and, where pectic enzymes are present, whether they have an invasive or a nutritional role or both. *C. m. michiganense* shows pectolytic activity on media of low pH suggesting PG rather than PL production. PG is produced by the opportunistic, non-fluorescent onion pathogen *P. cepacia*. This is in contrast to the fluorescent *P. marginalis* where, as in macergenic *Erwinia* spp., PL is the key enzyme in tissue maceration. When tests are made *in vitro* for the presence of pectic enzymes, the importance of a low pH for PG and a high pH for PL activity has sometimes been overlooked. Ability to rot potato tissue is often used as a test for macerating potential but (as with pectate gel liquefaction) it may not reflect pectic enzyme activity in other plant tissue.

Though *E. carotovora* is a major cause of spoilage of various vegetable crops after harvesting, opportunistic pathogens which produce pectic and other cell wall degrading enzymes are damaging too. They include *Pseudomonas* spp., *Bacillus subtilis* and *B. polymyxa* and *Clostridium* spp. (Lund, 1983).

Other cell wall degrading enzymes

Emphasis has been placed on pectic enzymes because they undoubtedly have a major role in certain bacterial and fungal diseases. But the same pathogens may produce other hydrolytic enzymes that promote invasion of cortical tissue or of xylem vessels. This is true of vascular wilt pathogens. Bacteria which attack monocotyledonous plants (which lack pectic substances in their cell walls) need other cell wall degrading enzymes (CWDE). Potentially significant CWDE include cellulases, galactanases, xylanases, arabanases and proteinases. Invading fungal pathogens produce CWDE in sequence (e.g. arabanases, xylanases, cellulases) suggesting that each substrate is exposed in turn. It seems that matrix rather than fibril degradation is most important in pathogenicity. Again, small enzyme molecules are the most effective. The bacterial pathogens in which CWDE are likely to have a role are macergenic *Erwinia* spp., *P. solanacearum* and some coryneforms such as *C. m. michiganense*. These enzymes play a part in some diseases caused by *X. campestris* pvs; they have been implicated only occasionaly in diseases caused by *P. syringae* pvs.

Toxins

Toxic substances produced by plant pathogens which are active at very low concentrations are, like plant growth regulators, of low molecular weight. This may facilitate movement in the apoplasm. They are often enzyme inhibitors but, unlike some fungal phytotoxins, none is host-specific. So far, only genes for the toxin coronatine appear to be plasmid-borne.

Toxin production appears to be confined to *P. syringae* pvs (Gross and Cody, 1985). These are pathogens of temperate crops so perhaps they need additional aids to promote rapid invasion at low temperatures. The toxins are commonly considered to be virulence rather than pathogenicity factors because some Tox^- strains can invade and multiply in host plant tissue and produce local lesions; the toxin appears necessary for full invasive capacity and typical symptom expression. Mitchell (1981) and Gross and Cody (1985) describe these toxins in detail and only selected features are outlined here.

Syringomycin This is produced by certain *P. syringae* pvs. It is a broad-spectrum biocide affecting a variety of plant, fungal and bacterial cells but sensitivity can vary widely. In plants, it may induce necrosis, chlorosis and water-soaking of tissue. Little is known of its chemical structure but it appears to have a peptide component. A related compound, syringotoxin, is produced only by pathovars that affect *Citrus* spp.

Coronatine This is produced by a *P. syringae* pathovar affecting grasses. The pathogen was previously referred to as *P. s. coronafaciens* but is now called *P. s. atropurpurea*. Confusingly, *P. s. coronafaciens* (which affects oats) produces tabtoxin, not coronatine. Coronatine may also be produced by *P. s. glycinea*. In plants, it induces chlorosis but its chemical nature is at present uncertain.

Phaseolotoxin This is produced only by *P. s. phaseolicola*. It induces large chlorotic haloes around the necrotic spots which give the disease its name, halo blight, and distinguish it from common blight caused by *X. c. phaseoli* in warmer climates. It is a tripeptide and moves through plant tissues; besides producing chlorosis, it retards growth and disrupts apical dominance. Halo formation is greatest at temperatures of 16–20°C and absent at 28°C. L-Ornithine accumulates in tissue because the toxin acts by inhibiting ornithine carbamoyl transferase (OCTase) which blocks the conversion of ornithine to citrulline and so blocks arginine synthesis. The toxin inhibits OCTase in a wide variety of plants and in bacteria, which means that *E. coli* can be used for its assay in the laboratory. It is thought to act by binding to active sites of the enzyme. Toxin production contributes significantly to the virulence of *P. s. phaseolicola* and may be essential for the persistence of this pathogen under field conditions; how it affects virulence remains unclear.

Tabtoxin This is a dipeptide produced by *P. s. tabaci*. Another pathogen on tobacco, *P. s. angulata*, is believed to be a non-toxigenic form of *P. s. tabaci*. Other *P. syringae* pvs are also thought to produce this toxin. It induces chlorotic and necrotic symptoms on infected leaves. The active component is probably a derivative of the dipeptide released by plant enzymes which acts by inhibiting glutamine synthetase (GS); this leads to the accumulation of ammonia. The process is enhanced by light and results in both chlorosis and necrosis. The overall consequences are very severe for affected plants. Tox^- mutants are sensitive to tabtoxin which should encourage maintenance of Tox^+ populations.

Other toxins Other toxins produced by some *P. syringae* pvs have been studied in less detail. It is likely that more remain to be discovered.

Other factors

Necrosis

Many necrogenic pathogens characteristically produce leaf spots or cankers (dead tissue). Blackening of tissues which follows cell death is usually associated with polyphenol oxidase activity and, for some pathogens, with tyrosinase. There is still much uncertainty about the early interactions between the pathogen and the plant cell and the ultimate causes of cell death. It is these necrogenic pathogens that, in incompatible interactions, induce the hypersensitive reaction (HR). This then raises the question, is a single agent involved in both cell death and HR? If so, why is cell death so rapid in the incompatible interaction and delayed in the compatible one? These questions are discussed further in Chapter 4.

E. amylovora is a good model because it does not appear to produce CWDE or toxins—the only obvious pathogenicity factors are EPS and a necrosis factor. As with various other necrogens, in the compatible interaction no changes in host cells are detected at first, even when pathogen populations are rising to high levels, but some leakage of water and ions occurs at an early stage. No agent unequivocably responsible for cell leakage has been isolated from pathogen cultures grown in artificial media.

In another system, *X. c. malvacearum* in cotton, membrane potential studies have suggested that an extracellular agent might not be necessary for induction of increased plant cell membrane permeability. With increasing populations of invading bacteria, the energy supply to the cells might prove inadequate to maintain both plant and pathogen cells. Alternatively, changes in nitrogen metabolism might lead to ammonia accumulation and a rise in intracellular pH above the optimum for proton-translocating ATPase activity in membranes in the dark (Novacky and Ullrich-Eberius, 1982).

Ammonia accumulation

Any rise in pH in plant tissues will seriously affect cell metabolism and the healthy plant must have means for regulating pH and for detoxifying ammonia, should it accumulate temporarily. Amides accumulate in diseased plants which might be a consequence of such a detoxifying process (Kosuge and Kimpel in Mount and Lacey, 1982). This may benefit the pathogen: increased disease severity has been reported when the amide asparagine was introduced into tissue affected by pepper soft rot (*E. carotovora*), fire blight (*E. amylovora*) and bacterial speck of tomato (*P. s. tomato*). In the last case it seemed probable that during the later stages of normal infection proteases of both bacterial and plant origin degraded plant proteins to amino compounds, in particular asparagine, and deamination then induced release of ammonia (Bashan *et al.*, 1986). Gaseous ammonia could then diffuse through plant tissue and damage cells beyond the infected area. As described earlier, tabtoxin is also associated with ammonia accumulation. Pectic lyases have a high optimal pH for activity so ammonia accumulation could benefit macergenic pathogens.

Ice-nucleating protein

An unusual virulence factors is the ice-nucleating protein found in walls of some cells of both pathogenic and saprophytic *P. syringae* pvs and in those of other leaf-surface colonizing saprophytic bacteria such as *E. herbicola*. Not all ice-nucleating bacteria are invasive pathogens. If, however, they induce cell death they are in a sense causing disease. The cell death is a result of ice crystal formation in soft tissue at temperatures above those where such crystals would normally form in plants and frost injury occurs at temperatures between 0 and −5°C. In pear and lilac, severe blossom blight can follow; two different *P. syringae* pvs are involved. The disease sometimes becomes progressive. In other cases, especially with herbaceous plants, young leaves are affected. Genes determining ice-nucleating ability can be deleted (see Chapter 6, Control).

Plant growth regulators

The plant growth regulators of main concern in relation to the diseases described in this book are cytokinins and the auxin indole acetic acid (IAA) which together promote cell division and cell enlargement, and ethylene (Kosuge and Kimpel in Mount and Lacey, 1982). IAA is a product of tryptophan and ethylene in methionine metabolism. Ethylene synthesis may be triggered by IAA and, in turn, ethylene stimulates synthesis of phenolic substances. Thus, any alteration in the normal balance of plant growth regulators induced by a pathogen is likely to affect the susceptibility or resistance of the plant to invasion by that pathogen. IAA is particularly important in barrier formation (See Chapter 4) as it stimulates mature plant cells to divide (de-differentiate).

No single role can be attributed to ethylene in either healthy or diseased plants. Many tissues can perceive and react quickly to small changes in ethylene concentration. Abnormal levels of ethylene are associated with senescence and with a variety of stresses apart from disease. Changes in plants associated with ethylene include: leaf epinasty and abscission, stem swelling, root proliferation and fruit ripening. At the cellular level, ethylene may induce leakage of electrolytes.

Some plant pathogens produce plant growth regulators *in vitro* but, *in vivo*, synthesis by the host plant may be of greater importance. For example, *P. solanacearum* produces both IAA and ethylene *in vitro* but it also induces changes in the shikimic acid pathway in the host plant leading to tryptophan accumulation; this would account for increases in IAA and ethylene production by the host plant. Whatever the origin of these growth regulators, many external and internal symptoms of vascular wilt disease are attributable to abnormal levels of IAA and ethylene (Buddenhagen and Kelman, 1964).

A. tumefaciens may produce low levels of plant growth regulators *in vitro* but transformed plant cells produce large amounts with the result that cells de-differentiate and uncontrolled proliferation is induced. This is the basis for plant callus tissue production in laboratory experiments and such transformed tissue has been cultured for 30 years without further intervention by bacteria or addition of growth regulators. In the case of *P. s. savastanoi*, which induces cell proliferation on olive, oleander and ash leaves and stems, this is due to IAA production by the invading pathogen. It is one of the few examples of a virulence factor that is plasmid determined. IAA^- mutants can still multiply in plant tissue but do not cause galls. *C. fascians*, the sole oncogenic coryneform bacterium, induces shoot proliferation and stem distortion. The pathogen produces cytokinins *in vitro*; it is not known whether the gene is plasmid borne.

A summary of suspected pathogenicity and virulence factors is shown in Table 6.

Table 6 Suspected pathogenicity and virulence factors

Pathogen	EPS	Necrosis	Pectic enzymes[a]	Low MW toxins	Growth regulators
E. amylovora	+[b]	+			
X. campestris pvs	+	+	(+)		
P. syringae pvs	+	+	(+)	(+)	1[c]
P. solanacearum	+	+	(+)		+
E. carotovora			+		
E. chrysanthemi			+		
Coryneform pathogens	+	(+)	(+)		1[c]
A. tumefaciens	(+)				+

[a] Many pathogens which produce pectic enzymes also produce xylanases, cellulases, proteinases or other cell wall degrading enzymes.
[b] +, major factor; (+), variable character or importance uncertain.
[c] Single pathovar or species (*P. s. savastanoi*; *C. fascians*).
[d] Production in host cells induced by the pathogen.
(EPS, extracellular polysaccharides; MW, molecular weight)

Agrobacterium tumefaciens

A. tumefaciens does not kill plant tissue so its overall strategy as a pathogen is described separately below. It induces tumour formation by transfer of plasmid DNA to preconditioned cells of host plants. Dicotyledonous plants are frequently affected but not the majority of monocotyledons; pectic polymers are rare in the latter (see Chapter 2) but their role in this disease is uncertain. In contrast to other diseases, where high populations of the pathogen are necessary for typical symptom expression, one cell of this pathogen can by transforming a single cell of the host plant induce host cell proliferation and gall formation—no subsequent action on the part of the bacterium is necessary. As with some virus diseases, tissue damage appears to be necessary for both entry and disease initiation but it is not clear why. One consequence of wounding is water-soaking of local tissue. This allows limited progression of the pathogen in intercellular spaces and while it persists is likely to favour bacterial multiplication and interaction between host and pathogen cells. Wounding will also induce host cell changes and release of signal compounds (see Chapter 4) which favour transfer of the tumour-inducing (Ti) plasmid DNA from the pathogen to the host cell. Cell damage might also expose attachment sites.

Evidence that attachment of the pathogen to the host plant cell is necessary is not completely conclusive. The suggestion that bacterial LPS and pectic polymers are involved has been questioned. It has been reported that plant protoplasts can be transformed only if they have begun to regenerate cell walls which suggests a need for interaction between plant cell wall components and the bacterium. The roles of EPS production and of cellulose fibril synthesis by the pathogen when in contact with plant tissue are unclear but the latter could help to maintain close contact between the pathogen and the host cell wall.

The mechanism of transfer of plasmid DNA from the bacterium to the plant cell is uncertain. Free DNA can be introduced directly into plant spheroplasts but is unlikely to survive in plant tissue. It is not certain whether the Ti-plasmid is transferred intact but only part becomes integrated in the host cell genome. It functions there as a plant gene and it has been suggested that at some time *A. tumefaciens* 'captured' some plant genes. The plasmid is a valuable vector for introducing other genes into plant cells. Such genes can be incorporated into the plasmid by transposon mutagenesis (see Chapter 5). There are now exciting developments in genetic engineering of plants using this system and other methods whereby DNA is introduced directly into plants

Another consequence of transformation is synthesis by the plant cell of unusual amino-acid derivatives, opines. Different opines are specified by different strains of the pathogen and may affect the morphology of the gall tissue. The pathogen can utilize the opines as sources of carbon, nitrogen and phosphorus which gives it an ecological advantage over other bacteria (which cannot utilize them) in the vicinity of the gall. A further advantage to the pathogen is that opines promote DNA transfer between Ti^+ and Ti^- strains of *A. tumefaciens* in the surrounding area. Plasmid genes also determine the host range of the pathogen and its sensitivity to the agrocin-producing strain of *A. tumefaciens* (see Chapter 6, Control).

Further reading

BASHAN, Y., OKAN, Y. and HENIS, Y. (1986). A possible role for proteases and deaminases in the development of bacterial speck disease in tomato caused by *Pseudomonas syringae* pv. *tomato. Physiological and Molecular Plant Pathology* 28: 15–31.

BRUBAKER, R. R. (1985). Mechanisms of bacterial virulence. *Annual Review of Microbiology* 39: 21–50.

BUDDENHAGEN, I. and KELMAN, A. (1964). Biological and physiological aspects of bacterial wilt caused by *Pseudomanas solanacearum. Annual Review of Phytopathology* 2: 203–30.

CHESSON, A. (1980). Maceration in relation to post-harvest handling and processing of plant material. *Journal of Applied Bacteriology* 48: 1–45.

COSTERTON, J. W., IRVIN, R. T. and CHENG, K. J. (1981). The bacterial glycocalyx in nature and disease. *Annual Review of Microbiology* 35 299–324.

EL-BANOBY, F. E. and RUDOLPH, K. (1979). Induction of water-soaking in plant leaves by extracellular polysaccharides from phytopathogenic pseudomonads and xanthomonads. *Physiological Plant Pathology* 15: 341–9.

GROSS, D. C. and CODY, Y. S. (1985). Mechanisms of plant pathogenesis by *Pseudomonas species. Canadian Journal of Microbiology* 31: 403–10.

HILDEBRAND, D. C. (1971). Pectate and pectin gels for differentiation of *Pseudomonas* spp. and other bacterial plant pathogens. *Phytopathology* 61: 1430–6.

MITCHELL, R. E., (1984). The relevance of non host-specific toxins in the expression of virulence by pathogens. *Annual Review of Phytopathology* 22: 215–45.

NESTER, E. W., GORDON, M. P, AMASINO, R. M. and YANOFSKY, M. F. (1984). Crown gall: a molecular and physiological analysis. *Annual Review of Plant Physiology* 35: 387–413.

OSMAN, S. F., FETT, W. F. and FISHMAN, M. L. (1986). Exopolysaccharides of the phytopathogen *Pseudomonas syringae* pv. *glycinea. Journal of Bacteriology* 166: 66–71.

SLADE, M. B. and TIFFIN, A. I. (1984). Biochemical and serological characterization of *Erwinia*. In: *Methods in Microbiology*, Vol. 15 (edited by T. Bergen). Academic Press, London, pp. 227–93.

SMITH, H. (1984). The biochemical challenge of microbial pathogenicity. *Journal of Applied Bacteriology* 57: 395–404.

SUTHERLAND, I. W. (1985). Biosynthesis and composition of Gram-negative bacterial extracelluar and wall polysaccharides. *Annual Review of Microbiology* 39: 243–70. (See also Sutherland, 1977, in Bibliography).

4 Pathogen invasion and plant responses

Experimental systems

Much of the work described here has been done with potted plants in greenhouses or in growth chambers varying temperature, light intensity, day length, humidity, soil moisture and nutrients.

Simple systems are essential where large numbers of cultures or mutant strains of bacteria need to be screened for pathogenicity. They are also valuable for the novice who wants to do simple plant-bacterium interaction experiments. Laboratory-grown plants and tissues include shoot cultures or young or germinating seedlings where primary leaves, cotyledons or hypocotyls are inoculated. Sometimes detached leaves or leaf discs are used for short-term experiments. For some diseases, tubers or immature fruits are useful and can be stored to ensure a regular supply of material.

More elaborate facilities are needed for callus, plant cell suspension and protoplast culture. Here the plant pathologist is at a disadvantage compared with the mammalian pathologist because plant protoplasts soon regenerate cell walls and monolayer tissue culture is not possible. The choice of test system often depends on resources. Ultimately, some findings must be tested on field crops.

Saprophytic bacteria are often included for comparison with pathogens but, surprisingly, common plant-associated bacteria such as *E. herbicola* and related non-pigmented epiphytes, *Enterobacter* and *Klebsiella* species or coryneform bacteria are rarely chosen. The most commonly used saprophyte is *P. fluorescens* but it is not always appreciated that this species name embraces strains of diverse origin (not necessarily plant associated) with different biochemical characteristics.

Invasion of plant tissue

Initial entry

Unlike certain fungi, bacteria have no means of penetrating plant surfaces. *A. tumefaciens* depends on a wound for entry and the same is often true for macergenic *Erwinia* spp. Invasion via natural openings is characteristic of most Gram-negative necrogenic pathogens and is associated with motility. In contrast coryneform pathogens, which frequently enter tissue via wounds (mechanical or nematode induced), are mostly non-motile, as is the insect-borne necrogen *E. stewartii*.

Necrogens Most necrogens can enter plants via natural openings such as points of root lateral emergence, water and air pores (e.g. stomata and lenticels) and secretory glands (e.g. hydathodes and nectarthodes)—see Fig. 6. A water continuum

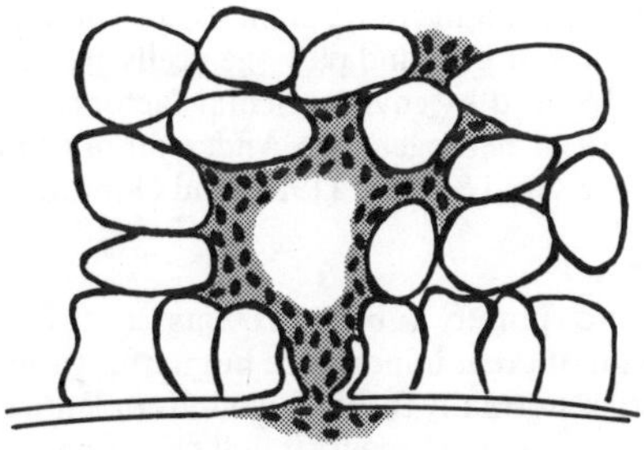

(a)

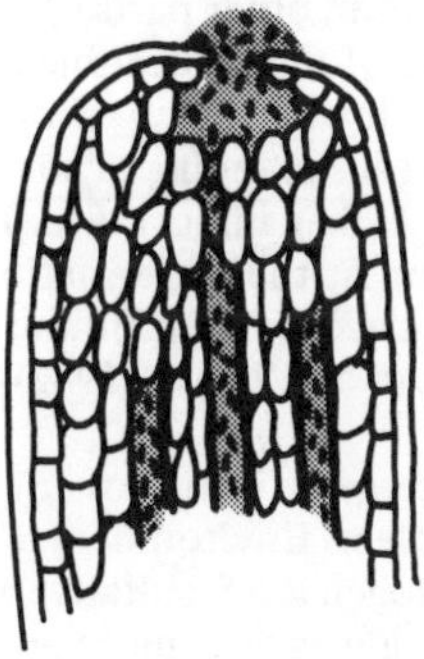

(b)

Fig. 6 Entry points for necrogenic pathogens. (a) Stomata: most are found on the lower surfaces of leaves; note colonization of substomatal cavity and start of invasion of mesophyll tissue. (b) Hydathodes: these occur at leaf margins; bacteria colonize tissue immediately below the opening and quickly reach xylem vessels.

between the outer and inner surfaces of the plant (most likely at night when there is rain) will aid entry via natural openings. Diseases caused by necrogens are normally most severe, however, when there is tissue damage during storms. Both wounding and wind-driven rain induce local water-soaking of plant tissue and the bacteria may be carried or move through tissue beyond the initial site of entry.

Some bacteria may colonize roots or aerial parts of plants near the entry site prior to invasion (see Chapter 6). It is possible that fimbriae have a role in aiding attachment to particular sites but this is still under investigation. Several pathogens show positive chemotaxis towards solutes excreted at leaf and root surfaces and towards nectar, but a connection with host specificity is suspected in only a few cases. Chemotaxis within plant tissue has not been demonstrated but free water would be necessary for movement.

As well as aiding entry of bacteria into plant tissue a storm can be a potent agent in the epidemic spread and establishment of many bacterial diseases. During a storm many different bacteria, both saprophytes and pathogens, will be spread between plants. Wind and hail damage will expose xylem vessels by snapping leaf veins or tearing off leaves and exposing leaf scars thus providing direct entry into stems. Cortical tissue will also be exposed and there will be temporary water-soaking. As a result a wide variety of bacteria may be sucked into xylem vessels, where there is negative pressure, and enter intercellular spaces between parenchyma cells. The question is, why do the great majority of these bacteria fail to colonize even the damaged tissue and only a very small minority produce a progressive disease?

At what point is resistance to incompatible pathogens first expressed in the plant? Leaf infiltration experiments indicate that in intercellular spaces this occurs at the surface of parenchyma cells. In the case of entry via hydathodes, studies with vascular necrogens such as *X. c. campestris* and *X. c. oryzae* suggest that resistance is expressed at the point of entry. With *X. c. campestris*, growth is equally good in xylem fluids from susceptible and resistant cultivars, indicating a cell surface reaction as in other parts of the leaf. On stigma surfaces, *E. amylovora* grows well on those of the susceptible host pear but not on those of the resistant cherry.

Following entry, many necrogens establish best in young plant tissue where cells are still expanding. The relative growth rates of host and pathogen cells are therefore of key importance. Both will be influenced by environmental factors.

For further information on initial entry of necrogens see Anderson in Mount and Lacey (1982), Billing in Rhodes-Roberts and Skinner (1982) and Goodman in Mount and Lacey (1982).

Macergens Entry of *E. carotovora* into potato tubers presents a different problem. Environmental factors are again of great importance but in this case the pathogen is a facultative anaerobe. Entry is normally through wounds or lenticels; bruising leads to more severe rots than cuts, possibly because it induces tissue water soaking. Dry lenticels are not vulnerable but when there is a surface film of water conditions become especially favourable for growth of the pathogen and for pectic enzyme activity and tissue is more susceptible. The water film ensures turgidity of cells in the lenticel area such that lenticels may enlarge and the thin layer of suberized cells break. In addition, oxygen depletion of underlying tissue may induce cell leakage and lead to further water soaking of tissue. This will allow motile cells of the pathogen to move in the cortical tissue. Under conditions of low oxygen tension the bacteria can still multiply and pectic enzyme synthesis and secretion is greatly stimulated (Maher and Kelman, 1983).

There may be a variety of reasons why maceration is inhibited when oxygen levels are high. Oxygen not only suppresses pectic enzyme synthesis, it also favours host tissue resistance reactions. If, following damage, oxygen levels are high the inert storage cells may become metabolically active, again favouring resistance responses.

Population dynamics

Most studies of population changes of bacteria in plant tissue involve infiltration of high doses of bacteria into leaf tissue. Results from different laboratories are not easy to compare because different systems and different cultures have been used. Nevertheless there is a trend and using a range of classic experiments a diagram has been constructed to illustrate the main points for discussion here (see Fig. 7). It is an idealized picture and should not be taken as representative of any one system. Gram-positive pathogens have rarely been studied in this way.

A *compatible* necrogen usually multiplies rapidly without lag; Sustained water-soaking of tissue makes little difference to multiplication rates or final populations. An *incompatible* necrogen may also multiply rapidly at first but will suddenly stop; it may (e.g. *P. solanacearum*) or may not die rapidly. Cessation of growth usually occurs at the time of plant cell death. In bean and soya bean the population levels may approach those of the compatible pathogen and equal them if there is sustained water soaking. At low inoculum levels however, the incompatible pathogen may multiple only slowly and not reach high levels; this may be closer to what usually happens under natural conditions.

If the tissue is kept water-soaked and in the dark, a saprophyte like *P. fluorescens* may multiply and produce necrosis but only at high starting doses. Thus only the compatible necrogen multiplies immediately and rapidly from low starting doses to reach high population levels (see Fig. 8). If it did not, it would be unlikely

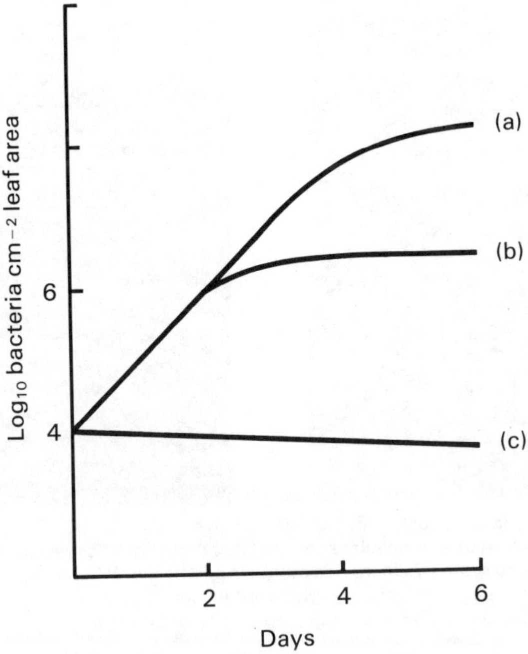

Fig. 7 Diagram to show contrasting population dynamics in leaf tissue of different types of pathogen and of non-pathogens: (a) Compatible necrogen; (b) incompatible necrogen; (c) macergen of non-pathogen. *Idealized representation* based on studies in dwarf beam (*Phaseolus*), soya bean and cotton at normal relative humidity levels. Where water congestion is maintained (in leaves other than those of soya bean), population dynamics of incompatible pathogens may closely resemble those of compatible pathogens and macergens; saprophytes will also multiply, sometimes reaching high population levels. When low doses of bacteria are infiltrated, population levels may decline more rapidly than shown. (For detailed findings see Ercolani and Crosse, 1966; Young, 1974a/b; Essenberg *et al.*, 1979; and Fett and Jones, 1984.)

to succeed. It would be interesting to know if the saprophytic bacteria so far studied are typical of all common non-pathogenic bacteria found on plant surfaces.

Disease progression

Most research has concentrated on the early stages of infection. Once established in the intercellular spaces between parenchyma cells or in xylem vessels, the pathogens, still have to contend with host counter-measures and questions arise concerning their progression in plant tissue. Some necrogens move rapidly in stem cortical tissue, sometimes in narrow channels between cells rather than on a broad front. Though some intercellular spaces are large, cells are often firmly joined by pectic substances. Not all pathogens produce pectic enzymes; conceivably, EPS binds calcium and weakens bonds. Perhaps the sheer pressure of bacterial growth

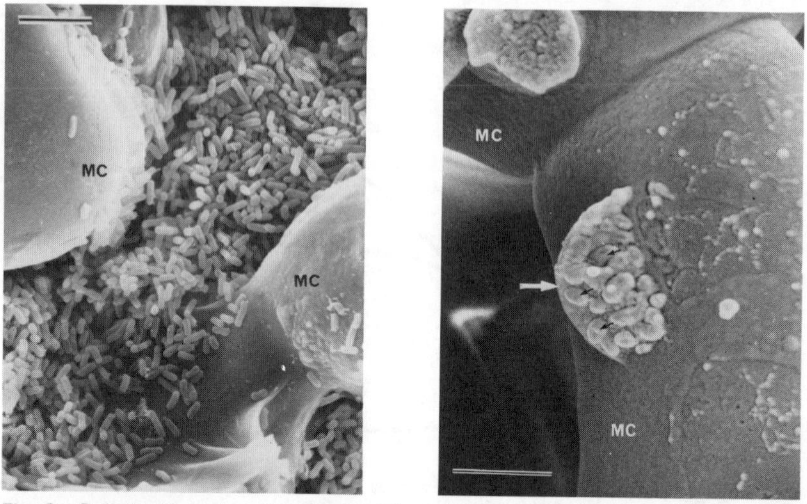

Fig. 8 Colonization of bean tissue (*Phaseolus vulgaris*) by *P. s. phaseolicola*. (a) Massive invasion of intercellular spaces of leaf mesophyll tissue. (b) A colony of the bacteria embedded in a polysaccharide matrix in pod tissue. MC, mesophyll cells. Bar = 5 μm. (Scanning electron micrographs reproduced by kind permission of J.W. Mansfield and I.R. Brown, Wye College, University of London.)

and EPS production enlarges spaces between cells. Other possibilities are that the pathogen induces changes in host cells which affect pectic polymers. Changes in the balance of plant growth regulators or ammonia accumulation might also be important. Toxin production by *P. s. syringae* pvs appears to increase invasive ability (see Chapter 3). A better understanding of mechanisms underlying disease progression could lead to better measures for disease control.

The progress of macergens is more easily explained. The pectic enzymes move in advance of the bacteria. *A. tumefaciens* does not need to invade tissue; once gall formation and opine synthesis have been induced the bacteria mutiply largely on the outer surface of the plant and in the surrounding soil. Hence, isolation of this pathogen from gall tissue often proves difficult.

Recognition and specificity

A few terms used in this and later chapters are worth defining. *Recognition*, the ability of a cell to discern differences, and *specificity*, distinctness or uniqueness, are terms that are widely but sometimes indiscriminately used. In immunology, recognition can also mean knowing again on second encounter. In this book the term *signal* is used for an agent that initiates an interaction and the receiver of the signal is termed the *receptor*. Where a characteristic response follows the interaction, the signal molecule is called an *inducer* or an *elicitor* Where necrogens produce a disease in their specific (homologous) host, the interactants and the interaction are called *compatible* and, in the opposite case, *incompatible*. In line with current convention a working hypothesis is called a *model*, though the term sometimes leaves the impression that more is known than is actually the case (see also Chapter 6).

In signal recognition, the receptor molecule is likely to be a protein; a single protein may carry more than one receptor site. Some proteins can change configuration and interact with other molecules so a receptor protein may also have a role in signal transfer via the membrane to intracellular organelles and the cytoplasm. Plant cell receptors involved in pathological interactions may have a normal physiological function which a pathogen can exploit. Whilst it seems reasonable to assume that plants have mechanisms for recognizing non-self molecules this has not yet been clearly demonstrated, though the hypersensitive reaction is usually considered to be a form of non-self recognition. It must not be forgotten that the pathogen itself is a signal receiver and the plant cell a signal producer. Current work suggests that certain constitutive plant phenolics can activate genes in *A. tumefaciens*. In pathological interactions, therefore, there may be a series of signal exchanges.

Models for responses to signal molecules in plant cells depend heavily on knowledge gained from mammalian systems (Clarke *et al.* in Roberts *et al.*, 1985). In plants there is the problem of how signals cross cell walls although plant growth regulators and toxins produced by plant pathogens are of low molecular weight.

Cell-cell binding

A. tumefaciens is the pathogen which would seem to have most need to bind to cell wall surfaces. Transfer of plasmid DNA presumably needs close cell-cell contact. However, it may be necessary for only a single cell to bind to induce gall formation. There is no doubt that bacteria of all types are frequently bound to plant surfaces including outer surfaces of root hairs and leaves as well as tissue cell walls. Recovery experiments and microscopic observations both demonstrate this. What remains uncertain is the nature of the binding, its specificity and its role in plant disease.

Binding can be a multi-step process. Initially it may be reversible, involving intermolecular forces such as ionic or hydrogen-bonding, calcium bridging or hydrophobic forces. In some cases the strength of the binding is reinforced by EPS production. Non-specific binding of this nature may be as important on outer surfaces of plants as it is in dental caries, which are also caused by bacteria (Marsh and Martin in *Aspects* 1, 1984). Both bacterial and plant cell wall surfaces carry a net negative charge and calcium bridging is a possibility. Fimbriate bacteria carry a lower negative charge and are more hydrophobic than non-fimbriate bacteria, allowing them to approach hydrophilic surfaces more closely than non-fimbriate types. In mammalian disease, some fimbriate pathogens bind specifically to certain mucous membrane surfaces. Mucous membranes are, however, outer surfaces of tissues. Binding in this way might be an advantage to a bacterium on the plant outer surface but not in intercellular spaces if it is to cause a progressive disease.

Non-specific binding is normally involved when plant products agglutinate bacteria, though some selectivity may be evident for lectins (sugar-binding proteins). Pectic polysaccharides and basic proteins have commonly been implicated. Avirulent mutants of *P. solanacearum* and *E. amylovora* which lack EPS are particularly prone to agglutination by basic proteins. Pueppke (1985) has reviewed critically past studies on binding of bacteria to plant surfaces and found conflicting reports and contradictory evidence but, as he points out, experimental difficulties make firm conclusions elusive.

Host specificity

Plant pathogens will have evolved alongside a specific host plant and its ancestors. Initially they may have lived saprophytically but then become plant adapted and, ultimately, adapted to a specific host. In the process they are likely to have become more and more dependent on their host and lost attributes necessary for a saprophytic existence, independent of the host plant.

Part of host specificity must lie in the ability of the pathogen to counter inhibitors produced by the host and to use what the host to offer, in the way it is offered, in order to reach rapidly high populations at appropriate times. But this is not enough. In necrogens it is evident that there is an interaction at an early stage between plant cells and the invading bacteria that determines whether or not the bacteria will survive and multiple for long enough to produce a progressive disease.

The nature of the molecules determining host specificity in the pathogen remains uncertain. Host specificity has to some extent been correlated with protein and fatty acid profiles, phage sensitivity and serological specificity (where protein or LPS molecules may be implicated) and with EPS composition (see Chapter 2) but these assessments may be too crude to give reliable results. Having identified molecules that determine host specificity it will still be necessary to determine their mode of action. When one host is attacked by several different pathogens, the basis for host specificity in each case will not necessarily be the same.

The limits of host specificity vary widely between pathogens. With some strains of *A tumefaciens* the range is narrow, with others it is wide. Of the macergens, many strains of *E. carotovora* have a wide host range but *E. c. atroseptica* is largely confined to potatoes. *E. chrysanthemi* tends to be host species specific. Necrogens often have a narrow host range but *P. solanacearum* varies; race 1 has a very wide host range, race 2 is confined to triploid bananas and race 3 to certain solanaceous plants (potato and tomato). *E. amylovora* affects rosaceous pip fruits (apple, pear and quince) and related ornamental trees and shrubs, including hawthorn, cotoneaster, pyracantha and *Sorbus* spp., but it does not cause disease in stone fruits and other rosaceous plants.

With *P. syringae* and *X. campestris* pvs, the host range is usually very narrow and may be confined to a few cultivars within a host plant species. The accelerated evolution produced by plant breeders may be matched by these pathogen (see Chapter 5). It seems possible with both *P. syringae* and *X. campestris* that a long period of evolution is not necessary for new pathogens to arise on new hosts.

Some pathogens show preference for certain organs such as flowers, leaves or roots. Some colonize xylem vessels in preference to cortical tissue. However, there is not the same degree of tissue specificity as it shown in bacterial diseases of mammals. Young tissue is more commonly invaded than mature tissue and the main need for the pathogen seems to be to obtain rapidly an adequate supply of water and nutrients.

Some plants are affected by a variety of pathogens, some by a few. An example of the former is the tomato which can suffer from canker (*C. m. michiganense*), crown gall (*A. tumefaciens*), various rots (*E. carotovora* and opportunistic *Pseud-*

omonas spp.), necrotic leaf and fruit spots (*P. s. tomato* and *X. c. vesicatoria*) and vascular wilt (*P. solanacearum*). Almost every tissue and organ is affected by one pathogen or another. So, like the dwarf bean, the tomato is a particularly useful candidate for comparative pathology.

Variability in pathogen and host

Different strains of a pathogen may vary in their ability to produce disease in a highly susceptible host plant, according to their degree of virulence. This will depend on a combination of characteristics including the ability to grow rapidly in host plant tissue at an early stage. Later, other attributes such as the production of particular enzymes or metabolites (including toxins and plant growth regulators) may influence rates of disease progression and the extent of damage to the host plant.

Different host plants will vary in their susceptibility to a particular pathogen for several reasons. First, this may depend on genotype. Sometimes a single gene makes the difference between complete susceptibility and complete resistance but often many genes are involved and intermediate responses may be seen. A second factor affecting the response of a host plant is tissue susceptibility. Growing tissue, where cells are still expanding in size, is often more susceptible than mature tissue; the overall nutritional and water status of the plant will also affect the response. Finally there are the the effects of environmental factors, including light, temperature and water relationships. These will affect both pathogen and host individually and the interaction between the two.

Plant responses to disease

Some of the components of the bacterial and plant cell interface are shown in Fig. 9. Unfortunately this tells us nothing of the molecular interactions that may rapidly occur between the cells. Healthy plants respond to stress and tissue damage in a variety of ways. Any stimulus at the plant cell surface can perturb the underlying membrane. Sometimes a simple physiological response will follow and any change will be reversible. At the other extreme there will be irreversible damage leading to plant cell death.

The consequences of plant cell death are many. Release of preformed compounds with potential antimicrobial activity has been described in Chapter 2. Of the other consequences described here it cannot be assumed that any are necessarily defence mechanisms against invading pathogens; many occur in response to stress or damage caused by a wide variety of physical, chemical or biological agents. There are, however, instances with some fungal diseases where a particular response appears to be invoked only by the pathogen. Whatever the nature of the host plant reaction, the most successful invaders are likely to be those that do *not* provoke host cell responses that would restrict their own growth or enzyme production during the early stages of invasion. Better still, they should induce responses that assist colonization.

Responses associated with cell death

Cell death due to pectic enzyme production by macergens has already been

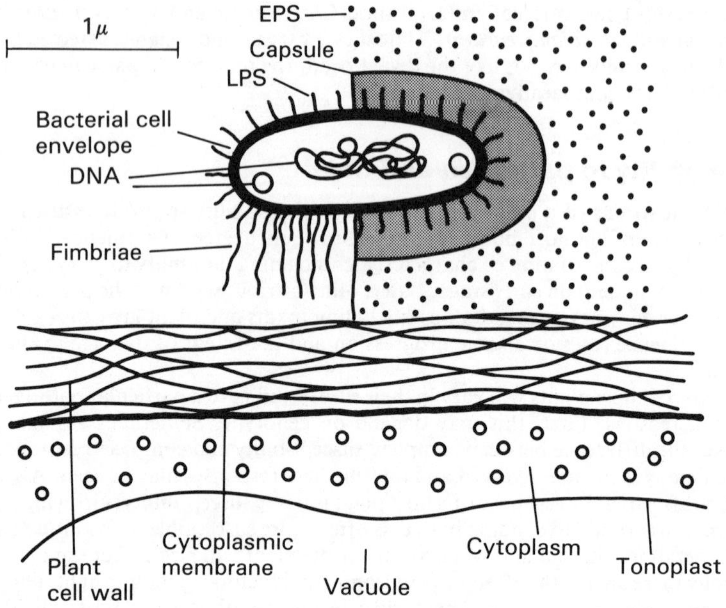

Fig. 9 Components of the bacterial and plant cell interface.

described (see Chapter 3). In the case of necrogens, cell death is characteristically delayed in compatible interactions but is often rapid in incompatible interactions (a pathogen in a non-host plant or a resistant cultivar of a host plant; or some avirulent mutants of pathogens in normal host plants). Rapid cell death is referred to as a hypersensitive reaction (HR) and is described in more detail at the end of this chapter.

Localized responses Apart from release of preformed cell constituents, plant cell damage or death is frequently associated with synthesis and accumulation of low-molecular-weight compounds from remote precursors in adjacent living cells. Some of these have antimicrobial activity and may also be toxic for plant cells themselves. Some workers prefer to use the term *stress metabolites* for such compounds regardless of the agent that induces them. Others use the term *phytoalexin* for all induced antimicrobial compounds, again regardless of the inducing agent. More commonly, phytoalexins are defined as low-molecular-weight antimicrobial compounds that are both synthesized by and accumulate in plants which have been exposed to microorganisms. The inducing agents (*elicitors*) used in experimental systems are of microbial or plant origin.

Much work on this topic has been concerned with fungal diseases (Bailey and Mansfield, 1981). There is evidence with some diseases that phytoalexins have an important role in plant resistance. In the case of bacterial diseases there are contradictory findings. Mansfield and Brown (1986) discuss the technical difficulties involved in evaluating the precise role of phytoalexins and the value of studying interactions at the single-cell level. The question of their relative importance compared with other consequences of plant cell death remains open. To play a major role, phytoalexins must be produced at a time, place and concentration sufficient to stop multiplication of a potential bacterial invader and they should be associated with genes controlling disease resistance. Phytoalexin accumulation is mostly associated with incompatible interactions involving necrogens where rapid plant cell death (HR) is induced. With compatible interactions plant cell death is delayed and phytoalexins do not accumulate. Pectic enzymes can also kill plant cells and induce phytoalexin accumulation but in soft rot diseases plant cell death in advance of colonization can mean that cells die too rapidly for induction of phytoalexin synthesis.

In incompatible interactions bacterial growth usually ceases at the time of plant cell death. Two questions arise: Would there have been time for adequate levels of phytoalexin to accumulate to explain abrupt cessation of bacterial growth? Are other consequences of plant cell death responsible rather than phytoalexin accumulation? Current studies at the single-cell level may help to answer such questions where multicellular approaches could not.

Phytoalexins are diverse substances and include classes of compounds found in healthy plants such as flavanoids, isoflavonoids, diterpenes, sesquiterpenes, polyacetylenes and stilbenes. Following induction, they accumulate in dead plant tissue. Because they are lipophilic and are not translocated, any protection they may give to the plant is localized to tissue adjacent to damaged cells. In tests *in vitro*, phytoalexins are usually more active against Gram-positive than Gram-negative bacteria but this may not reflect their activity in plant tissues.

Much interest has centred round phytoalexin elicitors. Many physical and chemical agents that damage plant cells are, in effect, elicitors but those of special interest are microbial and plant cell products (Darvill and Albersheim, 1984). Elicitors are presumed to activate expression of genes encoding enzymes required for phytoalexin synthesis. Recent work suggests that fragments of plant cell wall pectic polysaccharides can act as elicitors. These may be released by pectic enzymes of invading microorganisms or by plant enzymes activated by cell damage or death. Low-molecular-weight oligosaccharides from both plant and microbial sources are also believed to have a role in systemic responses to wounding and disease. Oligosaccharides may also have important regulatory functions in plants (Halvorson and Stacey, 1986).

Systemic responses There are many examples, particularly in cucumber and tobacco plants, where inoculation of a leaf with one pathogen (virus, fungus or bacterium) induces resistance in other leaves to infection by the same pathogen or certain other pathogens (Sequeira, 1983). Systemic resistance depends on the development of necrotic lesions by the pathogen introduced initially. The net effect in systemically protected leaves is increased protein synthesis. As with phytoalexins, any protective effect appears to be non-specific. Mechanical damage on tomato or potato leaves (such as that produced by chewing insects) also induces a systemic response in the form of proteinase inhibitor production by protected plant cells (Ryan in Kosuge and Nester, 1984).

The intensity of a systemic response appears to be related to the extent of plant cell death. Where the response is induced by wounding, crushing is more effective than cutting, perhaps because it releases higher levels of signal compounds. Where infection is involved, massive doses of bacterial inoculum or progressive invasion of tissue, which would provide a continual stimulus, give the best responses. There is still much to learn about the biochemistry of systemic induced-resistance responses. How inducing molecules, such as plant or pathogen oligosaccharides, are translocated is not clear. It has been suggested that they may produce localized effects which result in release of further signal molecules.

It has long been hoped that antimicrobial responses might be exploited to prevent or control plant diseases but they have not been demonstrated in all plants. They are not comparable to the immune response in mammals and may be short lived. Protection comparable to immunization in mammals is not likely. So far, the degree of protection provided has not proved adequate under field conditions but this research is still in its early stages. Not surprisingly, it is currently an area of intensive study. Potentials and limitations of induced resistance are discussed by Sequeira (1983). Better understanding of underlying mechanisms could be rewarding in understanding plant physiological processes as well as in crop protection.

Increased cell resistance and barrier formation

Calcium accumulation Damage and infections induce active metabolic processes in plants which lead to accumulation of cations, including calcium. Calcium pectate is not readily hydrolysed and walls become more resistant to pectic enzyme activity. Extracellular calcium may also have a role in the synthesis of phytoalexins and other agents involved in local and systemic resistance responses. It is also necessary for callose deposition.

Callose deposition Callose deposition is rapid at sites of stress and a shift in electrical potential can be enough to initiate callose synthesis. Polycations are potent inducers of callose synthesis. Like cellulose, callose is a glucan but the glucose units are β-(1,3) linked not β-(1,4). Callose is important in various ways apart from defence in plants and has roles in pollen maturation and tube growth and in pollen-stigma interactions, where it forms a seal in incompatible interactions. In damaged tissue, it can rapidly seal off injured cells and close connections that unite protoplasts of adjacent cells (e.g. plasmadesmata and phloem seive tube pores). At the cell surface, callose is deposited outside the cytoplasmic membrane.

The net effect of both calcium accumulation and callose deposition could reduce risks of plant cell damage in several ways. Where membrane damage is slight, osmotic stability might be restored.

Barrier formation Secondary thickening of cell walls has been described in Chapter 2. It will make plant surfaces less favourable for bacterial growth and for interaction between bacterial and plant cells and the thickened plant cell walls will be more resistant to degradation than primary plant cell walls. Hydroxyproline-rich glycoproteins accumulate in cell walls of damaged and diseased plants. Their synthesis may be increased in the presence of ethylene and they seem to be associated with lignin deposition.

More profound changes may separate damaged from healthy cells with formation of several layers of hydrophobic, suberized cells (Beckman, 1980). This process requires cell dedifferentiation (return to a state where they can once more divide). For this mature walls have to become plastic by removal of calcium. This must occur at a site beyond that at which barriers were formed at cell walls. One consequence of cell death, with accompanying release of phenolic substances and their oxidation, is the synthesis of the plant growth regulator IAA. IAA can travel through tissue and induce responses necessary for cell de-differentiation and renewed growth at a site removed from the necrotic area. The cells later re-differentiate and form the suberized protective layer.

In certain leaf spot diseases, such as cherry canker (*P. s. morsprunorum*), a few layers of suberized cells are formed and bounded by an abscission layer such that the necrotic area drops out leaving a 'shot hole' (see Fig. 1, Chapter 1). In this and other canker diseases of trees, damaged stem areas are walled off during the growing season to form well-defined cankers. Slow or inadequate barrier formation by a host plant may make it highly susceptible to progressive infection. The rate of barrier formation will depend on a combination of factors, including innate characteristics of the host, activities of the pathogen and environmental factors.

The hypersensitive reaction (HR)

In mammals, hypersensitivity (*not* known as HR) is an exaggerated or inappropriate immune response, usually associated with exposure to an antigen on second and subsequent occasions when specific antibody is present. It is a recognition response in the sense of 'knowing again' and may be associated with rapid and inflammatory reactions if the antigen enters the bloodstream immediately. Examples of hypersensitive responses are: various allergic reactions, including hay fever; severe reactions to bee venom or penicillin; blood transfusion reactions; delayed skin reactions to certain antigens. The immune system also has a role in another delayed reaction, tissue graft rejection. In plants too, tissue grafts may fail but there does not seem to be an immediate rejection reaction comparable to HR. There are other interactions in plants which, when underlying mechanisms are fully understood, may be relevant to plant-pathogen relationships. They include *Rhizobium*-room hair interactions in root nodule formation and pollen-stigma interactions in flower fertilization.

In plants, HR is characteristic of incompatible interactions involving Gram-negative necrogens. Some Gram-positive coryneform pathogens have also been described as HR inducers but this group has not yet been widely studied. In the case of macergens, pectic enzymes alone induce rapid cell death so that, where high doses of macergens are used, interpretation of results can be difficult.

An HR test is often used in diagnosis as a test for the pathogenic potential of necrogens when the specific host plant is not available. Because high doses of inoculum are used, HR can be mistaken by the inexperienced for a disease reaction and in the past, this led to erroneous reports of wide host ranges for some pathogens. The test for pathogenic potential has proved most useful for *P. syringae* pvs, *P. solanacearum* and *E. amylovora*. With *X. campestris* pvs, environmental conditions are critical.

HR test methods and responses

An outline of some features of the test follows; Klement gives a full account in Mount and Lacey (1982). Bacterial suspensions are usually infiltrated into intercellular spaces of plant tissue at high concentrations (10^7–10^9/ml). Suspensions may be introduced under vacuum or by pressure infiltration using syringes or pipettes. In fleshy tissue, a simple needle prick with inoculum from an agar culture may be satisfactory. Every method produces temporary local water-soaking of tissue. Tobacco leaves are widely used for the HR test because of their size and the ease with which they can be infiltrated; ten or more tests can be made in a single leaf and inocula can be introduced serially if desired. Leaves and other tissues of a variety of plant species are also suitable but reaction times may differ. Necrosis is usually evident within 12–24 h, in marked contrast to compatible interactions where signs of change may not be seen until 2–6 days after infiltration.

Following infiltration of the bacteria, the sequence of events can be divided into three stages. First, the *induction period* lasting about 3–4 h at the end of which the reaction is irreversible. There is then a delay, the *latent period*, before visible change in the structure of the plant cell is seen and there is leakage of electrolytes. This is soon followed by death of the plant cell and tissue collapse, the *necrotic stage*. With tobacco, this stage may be reached within 12 h when high doses of bacteria are used; it is followed by rapid tissue desiccation in the infiltrated area. In soya bean leaves it may be 24–48 h before the necrotic stage is reached and tissue collapse is less evident. Cell death is usually accompanied by browning of tissue due to oxidation of phenolic substances released from dying cells.

If low concentrations of bacteria are introduced into tissue there may be local cell death; there is evidence that a single bacterial cell is capable of killing a plant cell. Low-dose reactions may not be visible without the aid of a microscope; at most, small necrotic spots may be seen. Some strains of necrogen produce only necrotic spots, even when tested at high concentrations; the plant's response is usually delayed and accompanied by chlorosis. Chlorosis without necrosis may follow infiltration with non-HR inducing pathogens and saprophytic bacteria.

Factors affecting plant responses

Tissue characteristics and environmental factors can markedly affect responses and standardization of conditions is very important. In beans, the same strain of a pathogen may show disease development in young leaves and HR in mature ones. Higher temperatures (up to 36°C) favour HR in tobacco infected with *P. solanacearum* and *X. campestris* but not *P. syringae* pvs. Fleshy leaves or high humidity may delay HR expression. Maintenance of tissue water-soaking may prevent a typical HR response completely and even give the appearance of a compatible interaction in some leaves, but not those of soya bean. Conversely, low humidity may lead to suppression of typical tissue water-soaking in compatible interactions. Strains of some incompatible pathogens will induce only a slight reaction. Incompatible *X. campestris* pvs affecting cereal crops may give little or no reaction in either grain plants or dicotyledons. In spite of these reservations, with experience and standardization of conditions, clear distinction can often be made between compatible and incompatible strains of necrogenic pathogens in a given host plant and the test is widely used in research on plant-pathogen interactions.

HR induction

This is a major area of research and there are still many problems. Current work with fungal and bacterial pathogens seems to be getting closer to resolving some of these and attention is concentrating on substances produced by the pathogen when grown in association with plant cells, rather than those produced in culture media. It seems that the incompatible pathogen needs to be metabolically active to induce HR. Although the induction period is short, there is time for exchange of signals between plant and pathogen. So, the pathogen may be stimlated to synthesize a product not normally produced in artificial culture and the host cell may be changed in response to the presence of the pathogen. Membranes are very easily perturbed and cells are killed by a wide variety of agents. The problem is to find one agent (if only one is involved) that induces HR in the incompatible but not in the compatible host plant. In the case of one fungal pathogen, a low-molecular-weight basic polypeptide which appears to be such an agent has been isolated from infected tomato leaves (de Wit and Spikman, 1982).

Reactive oxygen species

During normal plant cell metabolism oxygen is incorporated into organic molecules and several reactive oxygen species are generated which are cytotoxic. They include hydrogen peroxide, superoxide, singlet oxygen and hydroxyl radicals; of these, the last two are the most toxic. In the intact plant cell a variety of protective systems prevent any detrimental effects.

Membranes are at particular risk from reactive peroxyl radicals that may be generated because membrane lipids contain a high proportion of unsaturated fatty acids, but enzymes, nucleic acids and pigments are also vulnerable. Lipid peroxidation, commonly implicated in membrane damage, may be induced in plant cells by a wide variety of stressful agents, including heavy-metal ions, air pollutants and wounding, as well as by viral, fungal an bacterial pathogens and their products. Bacterial cell membranes are also susceptible, so toxic oxygen species can be considered as components of plant tissue defence reactions which follow cell damage or death. In mammalian pathology, they appear to have a role in the death of bacterial cells following phagocytosis. The role of reactive oxygen species is currently an area of intensive study in plant physiology and pathology (Elstner, 1982).

Outstanding questions

It is still not clear whether necrogenic bacteria need to bind firmly to plant cell walls to induce HR. Whatever the mechanism of HR induction, it is not certain that the cytoplasmic membrane is the primary target; membranes of other cell organelles might also be involved. In a compatible interaction, leakage of electrolytes from plant cells is often induced at an early stage but the relationship between induction of this process and HR induction is uncertain. It is sometimes suggested that HR induction is suppressed in the compatible interaction and that capsulation and EPS production have a specific role in this suppression. Tissue water-soaking suppresses HR non-specificially and so tissue oxygen and plant growth regulator levels also require consideration. This is currently a fertile area for speculation and model building (Callow in Day and Jellis, 1986; Daly, 1984; Heath in Gould *et al.*, 1986; Keen in Ingram and Williams, 1982).

A summary based on current knowledge of postulated interactions between bacterial cells and plant cells and tissues is shown in Table 7.

Table 7 Summary of postulated interactions between bacterial cells and plant cells and tissues

Bacterial cell		Plant cell/tissue
Signals produced/received	↔ Interaction	Signals produced/received
A. tumefaciens (oncogen)		
Plasmid DNA transfer (plant wound necessary)	→	Cell proliferation Gall formation
External multiplication	←	Opine synthesis
Macergens		
Pectic enzyme synthesis (favoured by anaerobiosis)	→ PD[a]	Tissue maceration (wet rot) in advance of pathogen Rapid cell death, water retained, anaerobic so phytoalexins not synthesized
Rapid multiplication	←	
Compatible necrogens		
Signal/receptor suppression? HR suppression? Necrogenic agent? Extracellular polysaccharide Other products[b]	→ PD	Release of cell solutes but not inhibitors Water retained Slow cell death
Rapid multiplication	←	Phytoalexins not synthesized
Incompatible necrogens[c]		
Necrogenic agent?	→	Rapid cell death (HR)
Multiplication ceases Bacteria die (fast or slowly) Bacteria contained	←	Inhibitors released Phytoalexin synthesis No water retention Cell wall changes Barrier formation
Non-pathogens[d]		
No signal exchange?		No signal exchange? Inadequate nutrients?
No multiplication		Inadequate water? Preformed inhibitors?
Slow death of bacteria		Cell wall envelopes bacteria

[a] PD, progressive disease.
[b] Other products include toxins, growth regulators and hydrolytic enzymes, such as pectinases and proteinases.
[c] Some exceptions behave like non-pathogens.
[d] Saprophytes; oncogens or macergens in non-susceptible plant tissue; some incompatible necrogens.

Further reading

BAILEY, J. and MANSFIELD, J. (eds) (1981). *Phytoalexins*. Blackie and Son Ltd, Glasgow.

BECKMAN, C. H. (1980). Defences triggered by the invader: physical defences. In: *Plant Disease*, Vol. V (edited by J. G. Horsfall and E. B. Cowling). Academic Press, New York, pp. 225–45.

DALY, J. M. (1984). The role of recognition in plant disease. *Annual Review of Phytopathology* 22: 273–307.

DARVILL, A. G. and ALBERSHEIM, P. (1984). Phytoalexins and their elicitors. *Annual Review of Plant Physiology* 35: 243–75.

ELSTNER, E. F. (1982). Oxygen activation and oxygen toxicity. *Annual Review of Plant Physiology* 33: 73–96.

ERCOLANI, G. L. and CROSSE, J. E. (1966). The Growth of *Pseudomonas phaseolicola* and related plant pathogens *in vivo*. *Journal of General Microbiology* 45: 429–39.

ESSENBERG, M., CASON, E. T., HAMILTON, B., BRINKERHOFF, L. A. GHOLSON, R. K. and RICHARDSON, P. E. (1979). Single colonies of *Xanthomonas malvacearum* in susceptible and immune cotton leaves and the local resistant response to colonies in immune leaves. *Physiological Plant Pathology* 15: 53–68.

FETT, W. F. and JONES, S. B. (1984). Stress metabolite accumulation, bacterial growth and bacterial immobilization during host and non-host responses of soybean to bacteria. *Physiological Plant Pathology* 25: 277–96.

HALVORSON, L. J. and STACEY, G. (1986). Signal exchange in plant-microbe interactions. *Microbiological Reviews* 50: 193–225.

JONES, S. B. and FETT, W. F. (1985). Fate of *Xanthomonas campestris* infiltrated into soybean leaves: an ultra-structural study. *Phytopathology* 75: 733–41.

MAHER, E. A. and KELMAN, A. (1983). Oxygen status of potato tissue culture in relation to maceration by pectic enzymes of *Erwinia carotovora*. *Phytopathology* 73: 536–9.

MANSFIELD, J. W. and BROWN, I. R. (1986). The biology of interactions between plants and bacteria. In: *Biology and Molecular Biology of Plant-Pathogen Interactions* (edited by J. A. Bailey). Springer Verlag, Berlin, pp. 71–98.

PAVLOVKIN, J., NOVACKY, A. and ULLRICH-EBERIUS, C. I. (1986). Membrane potential changes during bacteria-induced hypersensitive reaction. *Physiological and Molecular Plant Pathology* 28: 125–35.

SEQUEIRA, L. (1983). Mechanisms of induced resistance in plants. *Annual Review of Microbiology* 37: 51–79.

DE WIT, P. J. G. M. and SPIKMAN, G. (1982). Evidence for the occurrence of race and cultivar specific elicitors of necrosis in intercellular fluids of compatible interactions of *Cladosporium fulvam* and tomato. *Physiological Plant Pathology* 21: 1–11.

YOUNG, J. M. (1974a). Development of bacterial populations *in vivo* in relation to plant pathogenicity. *New Zealand Journal of Agricultural Research* 17: 105–13.

YOUNG, J. M. (197b). Effect of water on bacterial multiplication in plant tissue. *New Zealand Journal of Agricultural Research* 17: 115–19.

5 Genetics of bacterial plant pathogens

Cultures of bacteria are not pure unchanging clones—mutants are sometimes inadvertently enriched so that colony variants (perhaps showing loss of virulence) arise. Colony variants of laboratory cultures *in vitro* have proved useful in genetic studies. Oblique transmitted light and the incorporation of dyes in agar media help to show up differences between colonies and sectors within colonies (Braun, 1966; Meynell and Meynell, 1970). Changes in cultures remind that both genotypic and phenotypic changes may also occur during the course of disease. In culture, loss of virulence (full pathogenic potential) of pathogens is common and reversion to virulence is rare but the possibility of reversion means that it is dangerous to use spontaneous avirulent mutants as biological control agents.

In the past, spontaneous mutants were supplemented by those selected for resistance to a variety of agents, including phages, bacteriocins, antisera and antibiotics. Physical and chemical mutagens, such as ultraviolet radiation, acridine dyes, nitrous acid and nitrosoguanidine (NTG), can be used to generate variants for selection. The problem with nearly all these mutagens is that, because mutuations occur at more than one site, several characters may be changed at once and reversions can occur. This is why transposon mutagenesis, where mutation at a single site is possible, is now so popular. Thus, with current techniques, safeguards against reversion are possible.

Loss of virulence is often associated with loss of particular phenotypic characters, such as production of EPS, pectic enzymes, toxins or other presumed key virulence factors. However, other undetected changes affecting virulence may occur simultaneously. With modern genetic techniques the equivalent of Koch's postulates can be applied to ensure that particular genes encode pathogenicity determinants. Also, it is now common practice to screen large numbers of mutants without prejudice as to the nature, product and function of a particular gene and unsuspected pathogenicity determinants may be revealed.

Barriers to communication are at present common because of seeming complexity which is sometimes more apparent than real. Those unfamiliar with plant breeding and/or techniques of gene manipulation need to have some background information in these areas of work.

Plant breeding

Some current genetic studies are based on strains (*races*) of *P. syringae* and *X. campestris* pvs, which can be distinguished by their interactions with different cultivars of their host plants (see Table 8). The picture is not as clear as shown because intermediate reactions can occur. Combinations of race and cultivar that give clear-cut results can be chosen and simple versions of the HR test can be used

Table 8 Host-pathogen interactions – simple examples to illustrate how new races of a necrogenic pathogen may arise

Host		Interactions with pathogen races (matching incompatibility gene)		
Cultivar	Resistance genes	1 (*A*)	2 (*B*)	3 (other/none)
Original	None	C[a]	C	C
New 1	A	I	C	C
2	B	C	I	C
3	A + B	I	I	C

[a] C, compatible interaction (disease); I, incompatible interaction (HR) which will occur when a resistance gene in the host is matched by an incompatibility gene in the pathogen e.g. A(*A*), B(*B*).
New cultivars arise through natural selection or breeding. A single gene change in the host (A or B) may induce resistance to an existing race of the pathogen; sometimes two or more genes may be involved (e.g. A + B). New races of the pathogen (2 and 3) may arise through mutation and overcome the resistance of a new cultivar.

for detection of incompatibility reactions but this simple approach is not applicable to all systems.

What is not certain is how far responses in race-cultivar systems are applicable in non-host systems where incompatible pathogens induce HR or where avirulent mutants do so in a host normally affected by the compatible wild-type pathogen. Some researchers believe that race-cultivar compatibility is distinct from these other systems. The relevance of findings in these systems to macergenic and oncogenic pathogens is also uncertain.

Concepts and terminology

Many of the concepts concerning the genetics of plant-pathogen interactions arose from attempts to breed disease-resistant plants. These concepts put emphasis on host resistance genes whereas mammalian pathology concentrates on disease resistance acquired as a result of exposure to a pathogen or its products and the intervention of the immune system. Concepts concerning the genetics of plant-pathogen interactions were initially based on fungal diseases, in particular, certain biotrophic (obligatory parasitic) pathogens. These concepts are now applied to both fungal and bacterial pathogens in general, sometimes without justification.

One of the basic concepts is Flor's gene-for-gene hypothesis which postulates that for each gene that conditions a reaction (such as resistance) in the host there is a corresponding gene in the pathogen. However, this suggests that the underlying mechanisms are simple and only takes account of clear cases of compatibility and incompatibility in race-cultivar interactions, not of intermediate reactions (Day, 1981). It has proved a valuable basis for research but in the process has generated a multiplicity of special terms, some of which are shown in Table 16 after the Glossary. Such terms (in particular the terms virulence and avirulence) have sometimes created a communication barrier between plant and mammalian pathologists, geneticists and others.

In plant breeding, resistant cultivars can be produced by introducing genes for resistance into previously susceptible cultivars. The pathogen that meets the gene product(s) responsible for resistance is now frustrated and referred to as 'avirulent' by breeders because the interaction between plant and pathogen is now one of incompatibility and HR may be induced. The term 'avirulent' only applies to that particular interaction; the pathogen has not changed (it has not *lost* a virulence factor) and is still 'virulent' (compatible) in the original cultivar. The incompatible response is considered to be a consequence of the presence of a 'gene for avirulence' (gene for incompatibility) in the pathogen. It follows that, because the pathogen is still virulent in the original cultivar, the gene for avirulence was present at the start and there must be other similar genes waiting to meet new genes for resistance in new cultivars. In some cases, the frustrated pathogen mutates and counters the resistance gene so that it becomes virulent (compatible) in that particular cultivar. A new race of the pathogen has thus emerged which, if competent in other respects, will counter the efforts of the plant breeder such that new resistant cultivars must be bred.

An extension of this concept is that, in race-cultivar interaction, specificity lies in the incompatible interaction and not in the compatible one (Ellingboe in Mount and Lacey, 1982). Not all plant pathologists are happy with the concepts or the terminology (Gracen, 1982) but they have been widely accepted. Daly (1984) discusses problems associated with current models of host-pathogen interactions. Current research seems to support these models but the findings may be open to other interpretations.

This outline does not do justice to current concepts which are built on wide experience of plant breeding and interactions in fungal diseases in particular. Its intention is to prepare the way for further reading in this area of research where genetic manipulation, alongside biological and biochemical approaches, may help to clarify some of the complex interactions involved.

One aim in current research is to isolate genes and gene products associated with HR induction. At the time of writing, neither an HR inducer nor a signal receptor on plant cell surfaces has been isolated and characterized. The possibility remains that HR depends not just on the interaction of single host and pathogen gene product but on a series of interactions and/or repression and activation of unsuspected genes in host and pathogen. It must not be forgotten that HR is also induced by pathogens in non-hosts and by avirulent mutants which have lost their pathogenic potential in the host susceptible to the original pathogen.

Gene manipulation

An outline of the ways in which bacterial genes can be manipulated follows. Additional information can be found in many other texts (for example Hardy in *Aspects* 4, 1986, p. 11). The techniques used are sophisticated but many of the principles are straightforward. Many of the miniaturized methods used in genetic studies and DNA analysis evolved from use of simple materials such as agar gels (electrophoresis), filter paper (chromatography) and velvet (replica plating).

Extrachromosomal DNA

Most of the genetic information in a bacterial cell is carried on a single chromosome with double-stranded DNA in a closed circular form. The DNA thread is about 1.0 mm long and occurs as a compact mass. When extracted *in vitro*, it can be cut into fragments by means of enzymes (*restriction endonucleases*). In addition, the bacterial cell may contain extrachromosomal DNA in several forms.

Plasmids are circles of DNA which replicate independently of chromosomes; the DNA can vary greatly in length. In gene manipulation, they are used to transfer DNA from donor to recipient cells. Some plasmids mediate their own transfer and may be used to mobilize other plasmids; some are involved in transfer of chromosomal DNA. Of particular value is the plasmid RP4 and its derivatives which allow DNA transfer between *E. coli* and many different Gram-negative bacteria. Plasmids carrying different antibiotic resistance genes as markers are useful for the detection and selection of plasmid-containing bacteria.

Transposons

Transposons (Tn) are transferable genetic elements that will insert into DNA molecules with which they have little or no base-sequence homology. They may insert randomly or at particular sequences or regions. They disrupt genes at the point of insertion and are, in effect, mutagens. Transposons may be excised precisely at low frequencies giving reversion. They may code for readily detectable phenotypic characters such as resistance to antibiotics and heavy metals, carbohydrate utilization, amino acid biosynthesis and pathogenicity determinants; some of these characters can be exploited in transposon mutagenesis. In addition, transposons carry genes for a transposonase (involved in transposition) and a repressor sequence.

Multiple antibiotic resistance can arise through accumulation and clustering on a plasmid of transposons carrying genes for resistance to different antibiotics. This means that selection for one gene for antibiotic resistance may result in selection for other closely linked resistance genes and may be a factor in survival of such genes in the absence of selection pressure (Hardy in *Aspects 4*, 1986). This is a major reason why use of medicinal antibiotics for control of plant diseases is looked on with disfavour (see Chapter 6). *Insertion sequences* (IS elements) may be associated with transposons; they are small and do little more than code for their own transposition but they can act as mutagens. Naturally occurring ones are suspected in *A. tumefaciens* and *P. savastanoi*.

Of the transposons available, Tn*5* has been used most commonly with plant pathogenic bacteria. It is a 5700 base pair element with a central segment that encodes kanamycin resistance and terminal IS elements that can move independently. Useful features of Tn*5* include: high transposition frequencies from vectors (see below) giving a high yield of mutant colonies; low insertion-site specificity so that mutations are randomly distributed in target DNA; comparatively stable mutants (if reversion does occur, antibiotic resistance is lost); and convenient restriction sites (where cuts are made) for mapping the location of Tn*5* within a target DNA molecule and for subcloning and sequencing the target DNA. Tn*5* mutagenesis is not applicable to all species of bacteria; even within one species the degree of success can vary between strains. Another mutagen is *phage Mu*. Unlike other temperate phages, Mu inserts into the bacterial chromosome for its lytic cycle. Like a transposon, it induces a mutation at the point of insertion, which occurs at a random site.

DNA transfer

The elements of methods of DNA transfer between cells are shown in Fig. 10.

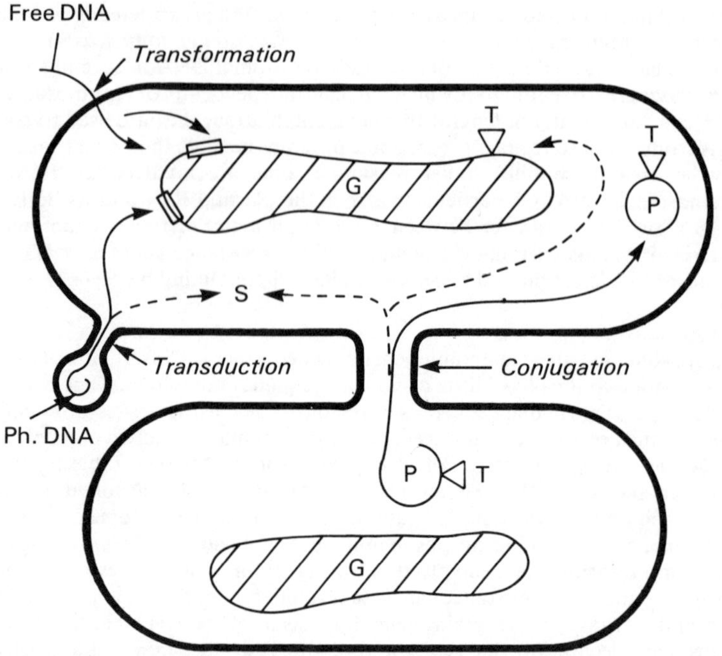

Fig. 10 The elements of methods of DNA transfer between cells. G, bacterial genome; P, plasmid; T, transposon; S, 'suicide' of vector; Fr, free DNA; Ph, phage DNA.

Vectors (carriers) are usually necessary for transfer of DNA between cells. However, small fragments of DNA may enter a bacterial cell without such aids and then integrate into the host cell genome; this is known as *transformation*. Certain temperate phages such as lambda (λ) and Mu have proved useful experimental vectors; the desired fragment of DNA is incorporated in the phage DNA and both are enclosed in phage protein coat. The DNA enters the recipient cell by the normal phage infection process, leaving the protein coat outside the cell. The DNA then integrates randomly (phage Mu) or at a particular locus (phage λ) on the genome; this is known as *transduction*. Some plasmids mediate their own transfer between cells by *conjugation* and are called *conjugative* plasmids. The DNA fragment of interest is incorporated in the plasmid DNA and transferred with it. The recipient cell is known as a *transconjugant* and the process of transfer as *mobilization*.

Plasmids are commonly used as delivery systems for transposons. A 'suicide' vector containing Tn*5* that has been used widely is pJB4JI; this code indicates that it involves a plasmid (p) number 4 isolated by J. Beringer (JB) at the John Innes Institute (JI).

Cosmid vectors combine the advantages of phages and plasmids and are useful for transfer of large DNA fragments. Plasmid DNA plus the desired DNA fragment are inserted into the phage genome and enclosed by the phage protein coat to produce a cosmid vector. Transfer is achieved by the normal phage infection process. The term cosmid arises from the fact that packaging of phage DNA depends on the presence of a *cos* site in the DNA which can be cut by a specific endonuclease. Use of a cosmid vector is implied in the terms *cosmid clone* and *cosmid library*. The hope is that, once the DNA has been transferred, the portion of interest should be incorporated into the bacterial genome. Replication of the vector is not always desired so some vectors are chosen for their inability to replicate in the recipient cell, hence the name *suicide vector*.

Recombinant DNA technology involves use of enzymes to cut DNA strands and join them with others to produce new combinations. The cutting agents, *restriction endonucleases*, act at different specific sites on the DNA molecule so that a variety of fragments can be obtained. A plasmid can be cut at a particular point and DNA from another source inserted. The DNA molecules are joined using *ligases*.

When a fragment of DNA has been incorporated in phage or plasmid DNA, multiple copies are produced by allowing the DNA to reproduce in a suitable microorganism (usually *E. coli*). A *clone* is a group of identical fragments of DNA. A complete genome may be cut into 1000 or more fragments each of which can be cloned in different *E. coli* cells. Such a collection is known as a recombinant plasmid or genomic *library*. A library of 500–1000 different *cosmid clones* can be maintained on one Petri dish. An outline strategy for the genetic study of virulence factors is shown in Fig. 11.

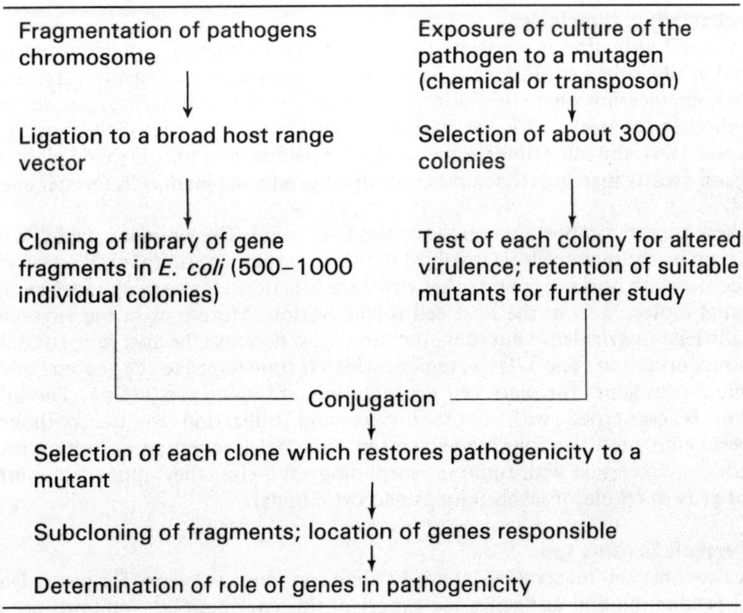

Fig. 11 Outline strategy for genetic study of virulence factors

Plasmids and pathogenicity

Much effort was put into the study of plasmids on the assumption that, like *A. tumefaciens* and certain mammalian pathogens, plasmids could carry important pathogenicity and virulence determinants. There are usually only 1–3 plasmids per plant pathogenic bacterium but up to 13 have been found in strains of *E. stewartii*, an insect-transmitted pathogen. As in other bacteria, plasmids may code for a wide variety of phenotypic characters, including heavy-metal and antibiotic resistance, but often no role for a plasmid can be found.

Plasmids appear to be associated with pathogenicity in some strains of *P. s. savastanoi* (coding for IAA production from tryptophan), some *P. syringae* pvs (coding for coronatine production) and *X. c. vesicatoria* (coding for incompatibility in a particular cultivar). Other reports need further substantiation (Panopolous and Peet, 1985). Plasmids are not longer believed to be involved in syringomycin production. Plasmids coding for heavy-metal resistance are found in *X. c. vesicatoria* (copper) and a *C. flaccumfaciens* pathovar (arsenite, arsonate and antimony). Pigment production and thiamine auxotrophy are plasmid-associated in *E. herbicola*.

Examples of genetic studies

Coryneform pathogens have received little attention because good genetic systems for their study have not yet been developed.

Agrobacterium tumefaciens

Crown-gall induction is associated with the large Ti (tumour-inducing) plasmid found in all virulent strains of the pathogen *A. tumefaciens*. It is a natural form of genetic engineering where the pathogen causes host plant cells to produce unusual metabolites (opines) which the pathogen can use as a source of nutrients (see Chapter 3). At the same time, induction by the pathogen of uncontrolled plant cell division greatly increases the number of opine-producing plant cells (Nester *et al.*, 1984).

There are three important regions on the Ti-plasmid. The *vir* region, which is not taken up by the plant cells, is involved in the early stages of tumour induction and concerned with host range and other virulence functions. Some of its genes require a signal molecule from the host cell for activation. Mutations in the *vir* region usually lead to avirulence but they sometimes just decrease the host range or delay tumour formation. The T-DNA region, which is transferred to the genome of the plant, carries genes for plant cell proliferation and opine production. The third region is concerned with opine uptake and utilization by the pathogen. Experimental modifications made by insertion or deletion mutagenesis have identified loci concerned with tumour morphology and size; they appear to control plant growth regulator levels (auxins and cytokinins).

Macergenic *Erwinia* spp.

To cause host cell maceration, these *Erwinia* spp. need *pel* genes for pectic lyase (PL) production and *out* genes for export of this enzyme. *Out*$^-$ mutants are no longer pathogenic because the enzyme accumulates in the periplasmic space. Whilst each strain may have several PL isozymes coded for by different genes, genetic studies have shown that *endo*-enzymes active at high pH values are the most destructive.

Several questions arise which may soon be answered as a result of current intensive studies. Is PL production all that is necessary for macergenic pathogenicity? Can *E. coli* be made pathogenic simply by transferring PL genes? Is PL production necessary for growth of the pathogen in tissue? Are additional genes necessary, for example genes for initiation of infection by low numbers of bacteria, for full virulence or for the limited host specifity observed in some members of this group? *Pel* genes have been cloned in and expressed by *E. coli* but the resultant bacterium is not a competent pathogen, partly because it lacks *out* genes such that the enzyme accumulates in the periplasmic space. Independent evident suggests that macergenic *Erwina* spp. (but not *E. coli*) multiply in plant tissue before maceration but for progressive disease it seems likely that both water and nutrients supplied by the maceration process are necessary.

Pectic enzyme regulation has been studied by cloning and characterizing PL and other pectic enzyme genes. Further detail will be obtained with the aid of mutants. Also, study of factors controlling enzyme export is now possible (Collmer and Keen 1986).

Necrogenic pathogens

Staskawicz *et al.* (1984) have transferred a gene determining incompatibility between races of *P. s. glycinea*. A genomic DNA library of *P. s. glycinea* race 6 in *E. coli* was constructed and 680 random DNA clones were mobilized in individual conjugations with race 5 strains of the pathogen. One of these clones changed race 5 from compatible to incompatible in host plant cultivars normally susceptible to race 5 and resistant to race 6 (see Table 9). The same clone also changed race I and race 4 strains in the same way but when it was transferred to the non-pathogens *P. fluorescens*, *Rhizobium japonicum* and *E. coli* it did not change them into HR inducers. Change from incompatibility to compatibility was never observed. The clone was mapped and two adjacent DNA fragments were identified as important in the determination of race specificity; they appear to code for a protein but this is not necessarily the HR-inducing molecule.

Whilst these findings appear to be consistent with the pathogen 'avirulence' gene concept, there is little information on the genetics of the host plant. Experience with other systems (Crute, 1986) suggests that two or more genes may be involved in host resistance. On theoretical grounds there might be three in the soya bean system.

Table 9 Transfer of genes associated with incompatibility in *P. s. glycinea*

P. s. glycinea race	Interaction in soya bean cultivar[a]						
	He	F	N	P	Hy	A	C
6	C	C	C	I	I	I	I
5	C	I	I	C → I	C → I	I	I
1	I	C	I	C → I	I	C → I	I
4	C	C	C	C → I	C → I	C → I	C → I

[a] C, compatible; I, incompatible; C → I, change when gene clone from race 6 was transferred to races 5, 1 and 4.
(Based on data of Staskawicz *et al.*, 1984.)

Genes for ice-nucleation activity in both *P. s. syringae* and *E. herbicola* have been cloned. In both, the activity was expressed well in the strain of *E. coli* used to construct the genome library.

Some strains of *X. c. vesicatoria* (race 2) harbour plasmids with loci for both copper resistance and incompatibility in certain pepper cultivars. The plasmid is self-transmissible and has been introduced into race 1 strains (copper sensitive, compatible), which then became simultaneously copper resistant and incompatible in the originally susceptible cultivar. Race 2 changes spontaneously to race 1 at a high frequency (4×10^{-4} per cell per division) but this does not appear to be associated with loss of the plasmid (Stall *et al.*, 1986).

In *X. c. campestris*, a cosmid clone restores pathogenicity in a chemical induced mutant which is defective in secreting extracellular protease and pectic lyase (PL); both enzyme activities are restored to the wild-type level (Daniels in Day and Jellis, 1986). DNA segments which restore pathogenicity have been cloned from several other pathogens including *E. amylovora*, macergenic *Erwinia* spp. (mutants with enzyme secretion defects), *E. stewartii*, *P. s. phaseolicola* (mutants with altered toxin production), *P. s. pisi*, and *P. solanacearum*.

Some preliminary non-genetic experiments with *E. amylovora* were made using colony variants and phage-resistant avirulent mutants that were EPS^- but still induced HR (Bennett, cited by Billing, 1984). An avirulent EPS^+, HR^- strain was also available. Though alone neither produced typical symptoms (copious ooze) on immature pear slices, when HR^+, EPS^- strains (but not HR^-, EPS^- strains) were mixed individually with the EPS^+, HR^- strain, typical symptoms were produced. This suggests that HR-inducing ability is a pathogenicity factor. Indirect evidence (including galactose sensitivity) suggested that inability to synthesize EPS (primarily a galactan) was due to lack of the enzyme. UDP-gal-4-epimerase in the phage-resistant mutants (Billing, 1984). Studies of genetics and biochemistry of this enzyme have been well studied in *E. coli* and Salmonella LPS synthesis and preliminary reports of genetic studies of the enzyme on *E. stewartii* (Coplin and co-workers) support the suggested role of this enzyme in EPS production.

In current genetic studies with *E. amylovora* (Beer and co-workers), mutants with altered pathogenicity have been obtained, some of which have altered HR-inducing ability. This suggests that HR-inducing ability is essential for pathogenicity. Perhaps further genetic studies will clarify the separate and combined roles of HR-inducing ability and EPS production in pathogenicity.

These are just some examples of current findings. With the considerable research effort currently being invested in genetic studies, the full impact and significance of this work should soon emerge.

Further reading

BILLING, E. (1984). Studies on avirulent strains of *Erwinia amylovora*. *Acta Horticulturae* 151: 249–53.

BRAUN, W. (1966) *Bacterial Genetics* , 2nd ed. W. B. Saunders Co., Philadelphia.

CHATTERJEE, A. K. and VIDAVER, A. K. (1986). Genetics of pathogenicity factors: application to phytopathogenic bacteria. *Advances in Plant Pathology*, Vol. 4 (edited by D. S. Ingram and P. H. Williams). Academic Press, London and Orlando, Florida.

COLLMER, A. and KEEN, N. T. (1986). The role of pectic enzymes in plant pathogenesis. *Annual Review of Plant Pathology* 24: 383–409.

CRUTE, I. R. (1986). Investigations of gene-for-gene relationships; the need for genetic analyses of both host and parasite. *Plant Pathology* 35: 15–17.
DALY, J. M. (1984). The role of recognition in plant disease. *Annual Review of Phytopathology* 22: 273–307.
DAY, P. R. (1981). Genetics of pathogenic fungi. In: *Genetics as a Tool in Microbiology* (edited by S. W. Glover and D. A. Hopwood). Cambridge University Press, Cambridge, pp. 361–78.
GRACEN, V. E. (1982). Role of genetics in etiological phytopathology. *Annual Review of Phytopathology* 20: 219–33.
MILLS, D. (1985). Transposon mutagenesis and its potential for studying virulence genes in plant pathogens. *Annual Review of Phytopathology* 23: 297–320.
NESTER, E. W. and KOSUGE, T. (1981). Plasmids specifying plant hyperplasias. *Annual Review of Microbiology* 35: 531–65.

6 Epidemiology and disease control

Epidemiology

A thorough understanding of the biology and epidemiology of each bacterial disease is an essential preliminary to the assessment of risks and to control. Mistaken assumptions can lead to time-wasting efforts. A valuable source of information on bacterial diseases is often found in advisory leaflets published by government departments of agriculture in different countries. It is worth comparing and contrasting here the characteristics of a few common bacterial diseases.

Black leg This disease of potato is caused by the macergen *E. c. atroseptica* and is important in temperate climates. All macergenic *Erwinia* spp. can infect potato but *E. c. atroseptica* grows well at low temperatures (15°C, optimum about 20°C). Black leg is often worst in wet soils and in cool wet summers. The pathogen is carried on seed potatoes and lesions usually occur at the base of stems near decaying tubers. Xylem vessels are commonly invaded and stems may be colonized without showing signs of disease. Some aerial spread of the pathogen can occur late in the growing season, so contamination of disease-free crops from outside sources is likely. Also, towards the end of the season, bacteria from diseased plants are washed into the soil and contaminate new tubers.

Fire blight This disease of pears and related trees and shrubs (woody plants) is caused by *E. amylovora* which is a necrogen. The pathogen overwinters mostly in cankers on small twigs or main stems. Rain spreads bacteria from such sources in

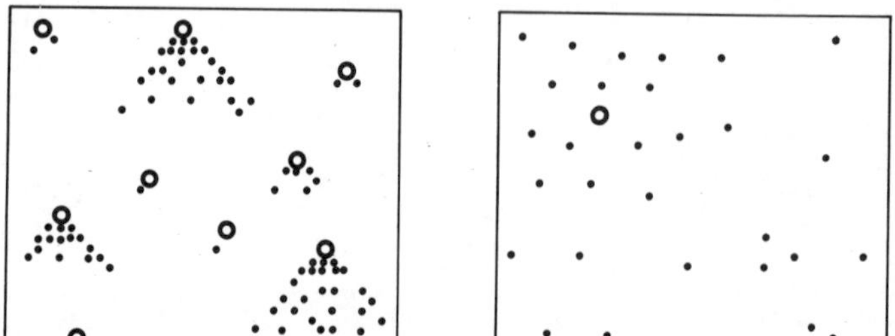

(a) (b)

Fig. 12 Patterns of disease spread: (a) spread from several foci by wind-blown rain during a storm, when leaf water-soaking and damage is likely (b) spread between flowering trees by bees from a single focus (*E. amylovora*).

spring but pollinating insects, especially bees, are responsible for much of the spread of the disease between trees during bloom (see Fig. 12). Wind-blown rain during damaging storms can also be important in spreading disease and encourages infection of young shoots.

The pathogen moves primarily in cortical tissue. If it enters xylem vessels it must escape to produce typical progressive disease. Though infection and some progression may occur at temperatures below 18°C, severe pear blossom blight is only seen in warm weather (21–30°C), which is rare during bloom in northern climates. Hosts vary widely in susceptibility. At one extreme, a canker may form and progression cease at the base of a blossom cluster; at the other, a young tree may be invaded from top to bottom and killed in a single season. Sale of unsuspected infected plants is a major cause of spread within and between countries (see *cryptic* infections, later in this chapter).

Halo blight Halo blight of beans (caused by *P. s. phaseolicola*, a necrogen) is initially seed borne but spread occurs between plants as the season progresses, particularly during storms (see Fig. 12). which encourage stomatal invasion. Both xylem vessels and cortical tissue are invaded, which is unusual since most *P. syringae* pvs primarily colonize cortical tissue. Seeds may be contaminated internally through invasion or externally during harvesting of infected plants. A valuable comparative study of the histology of three bean blights, caused by *P. s. phaseolicola*, *X. c. phaseoli* and *C. flaccumfaciens* was made by Zaumeyer (1932).

Black rot This disease in crucifers (caused by *X. c. campestris*, a necrogen) is also seed borne but xylem vessels are preferentially invaded following infection via hydathodes. The disease may spread systemically or remain as limited marginal chlorotic lesions with blackened veins. As with black leg and halo blight, the pathogen may overwinter in soil in association with diseased plant tissue.

Crown gall The pathogen (*A. tumefaciens*, an oncogen) persists in the soil but not in association with plant debris. It usually enters through wounds near the soil surface but plant tissue is not normally invaded beyond the point of entry and initial water-soaked area, nor is it killed. In cane galls and vines, aerial galls may be found and movement in the vascular system is a possibility; wounding in such cases may be due to frost damage. Infection of stone-fruit trees and roses commonly occurs in nurseries and control measures centre round immediate protection of cuttings and young plants subject to damage during handling.

Though the epidemiology of each disease has unique features, some features are common to many. Spread of disease is often favoured by wind-blown rain and epidemic disease is often associated with damaging storms. Infected plant debris may remain a source of inoculum in soil but on the soil surface there is also the chance of dry wind dispersal. Disease development is usually maximal in the temperature range 18–30°C.

There is a common assumption that bacterial disease is favoured by humid weather. This is partly true but rainfall is the key weather factor. Rain leads to a high soil moisture content and hence high plant cell turgor; it favours disease

Table 10 Means of survival of pathogens during the dormant season (overwintering)

Soil:	plant debris, roots (host or non-host)
Plants:	stem cankers, leaf scars, buds, fruits, tubers, seeds; alternative hosts, non-hosts
Invertebrates:	insects, nematodes

Table 11 Agents for spread of bacteria

Plant material:	seeds, cuttings, tubers, fruits, bud or graft-wood, whole plants
Machinery and tools:	cultivating and spray equipment, pruning knives, secateurs, saws
Water:	rain splash, wind-driven rain, irrigation.
Wind:	aerosols, strands, insects
Insects and birds:	pollination, damage

dissemination and entry into plant tissue and encourages tissue water soaking. Irrigation is not entirely equivalent to rain but overhead irrigation can be a potent factor in spreading disease and in maintaining leaf-surface wetness.

Summaries of means of survival of pathogens during the dormant season (overwintering) and of ways in which they may be spread are shown in Tables 10 and 11.

Plant surface colonization

The ease with which pathogens can be isolated from plant surfaces varies widely. Some pathogens rarely colonize plants surfaces, others are only found in association with their host, and some colonize a variety of weeds or crop plants. Survival in soil for long periods sometimes occurs around roots of growing plants (for example *P. solanacearum* on both host and non-host plants) but usually only in association with plant debris (for example *E. carotovora* and *X. campestris* pvs)

A detailed discussion of epiphytic colonization is outside the scope of this book (see Blakeman in Mount and Lacey, 1982) but the terms *epiphytic phase*, *latent infection* and *cryptic infection* need explanation. When plant surfaces are moist or the relative humidity is high, some pathogens multiply saprophytically for short or long periods on host plant surfaces, including roots (*P. solanacearum*), leaves (*P. syringae* and some of its pathovars) and stigmas and blossom cups (*E. amylovora*). On leaves it is not clear to what extent pathogens multiply on the surface, which will often be dry, and to what extent they multiply in substomatal cavities or small wounds and abrasions. Not all multiplication will induce plant cell death and not all cell death is visible to the naked eye.

The stigma surface is very different from that of the leaf; it is moist and concentrations of nutrients are higher. This encourages multiplication of a variety of saprophytes, including fluorescent pseudomonads and *E. amylovora* (Thomson, 1986). Nectar secreted in the blossom cup provides a good medium for the multiplication of both saprophytic and pathogenic bacteria. Where pathogens have an epiphytic phase, high bacterial populations will mean greater chances of infection when environmental conditions become favourable (perhaps during a storm); or, in the case of fire blight, greater chances of blossom to blossom spread by bees.

When bacteria are isolated from leaf or flower washings, it is not possible to distinguish those which have been multiplying saprophytically and those which have initiated disease but have not reached high enough numbers to produce typical symptoms. In some cases these may prove to be *latent* infections which will progress when environmental conditions become favourable; in others there will be no progress because the plant tissue has matured and is no longer susceptible to infection. *Cryptic* (hidden) infection is where a necrotic lesion is present but not visible to the naked eye or indistinguishable from damage due to other causes. When epiphytic populations are estimated they may include bacteria from such sources.

Another form of cryptic infection occurs with fire blight when wind or hail expose xylem vessels through damage or leaf detachment. Bacteria may be sucked in because of negative pressure in the vessels but will be unable to escape from the mature vessels. They may multiply for a while and produce blackening of dead cells (visible when stems are dissected) but fail to produce a progressive disease. Thus, seemingly healthy stems may be carrying a significant amount of inoculum, which can escape only if the stems are cut or broken. This means that, when examining dormants buds on trees for signs of colonization by the pathogen (as opposed to surface contamination), care must be taken to exclude leaf scar tissue.

Disease risk assessment

Assessment of risks of outbreaks of disease and of epidemics requires more than daily weather records. It needs sound knowledge of the natural history of the disease and as much information on field conditions can be reasonably, be recorded. It is always worth attempting risk assessment, even though precision is often low, because it is certain to lead to a better understanding of the disease and better prospects for its control.

Epidemic modelling is more commonly attempted with fungal than with bacterial plant diseases. In some respects fungal diseases are easier to handle. They are also often of greater economic importance than bacterial diseases. Inoculum potential can be more easily assessed and there are usually fewer variables to consider in relation to spread and risk of infection. With fungal diseases routine spraying of control agents is common and economy in their use through risk assessment is needed. Teng (1985) sums up the present position; accurate simulation of plant diseases may be a long way off in most cases. A major reason for this is imperfect and incomplete data; also, data cannot always be presented in a precise, quantitative fashion.

Some epidemic models are referred to as predictive systems. This can be misleading if they rely on weather yet to come. They may however predict that, because of high risks of infection or following a damaging storm, trouble is likely if potential inoculum was present at the time. A model might indicate that build up of potential inoculum probably occurred before the storm. It might also indicate, given certain field factors, which plantations are most risk. A model used on a day-to-day basis could then help to predict when symptoms might be evident, i.e. the disease development period.

Among bacterial diseases, fire blight has received more attention than most with regard to risk assessment. As shown earlier, its natural history is not simple. Table 12 shows some of the information that should, ideally, form part of any model.

Table 12 Some field factors used (alongside daily meteorological records) in fire blight risk assessment

Host phenology:	flowering and shoot growth periods
Host susceptibility:	cultivar, age, cultural factors
Number of susceptible targets;	blossoms, shoots
Risk of damage:	storms, insects
Risk of inoculum spread:	rain, wind, insects
Inoculum potential:	past and current infections
Alternative hosts:	e.g. hawthorn, cotoneaster

The list is formidable; even with good records, the inoculum potential and number of targets at risk at any one time are not easy to assess. Nevertheless, efforts have been rewarding enough to sustain attempts to increase the accuracy in assessing risks in different climatic areas, timing spray applications and timing searches for signs of new outbreaks of disease. As a supplement to local knowledge and experience, simple models can be of great value. Often it is enough to record daily maximum and minimum temperatures, daily rainfall and the occurrence of damaging storms in the locality. Evaluation of storm damage means looking at the affected crop and can only be done at the local level. Precision cannot be expected where judgements are based on weather records alone.

Disease control

Why have bacterial plant diseases in general proved so difficult to control? Success with crown gall control is a special case and not necessarily a good model for the control of other bacterial plant diseases. Lack of success with other diseases is partly a matter of low investment in research because of the relatively low economic importance of bacterial diseases compared with fungal and viral diseases of plants. Yet crop lossess in the field and during storage are high and rewards for good bacterial disease control could be great. In recent years prospects for new chemical control agents have diminished because of the high costs of development which have to be met by sales. Added to this is the increased resistance by the public to chemical sprays. There may well be orphan compounds (potentially effective but not developed) on the shelves now but there are few available for trial at present.

There are also intrinsic factors peculiar to bacterial plant diseases which make control difficult. Plants have only a primitive circulation system to aid systemic movement of a control agent and consequently the agent may not reach sites where the pathogen persists. Plants have no immune system to back up what control is achieved and control agents need to be applied every season. Because the plant, in its most susceptible state, is continually growing and producing new, unprotected tissue, repeated applications of a protective agent may be necessary during periods of high risk of infection. Many bacterial pathogens spend little time on plant surfaces and may not easily be controlled by surface sprays. Many potential control agents have little penetrative power and phytotoxicity precludes the use of some.

Bacteria are very different biologically from fungi, which may have in their life cycle a vulnerable period which can be broken, for example, during spore germination or tissue penetration. Furthermore, bacteria tend to grown more rapidly and are not susceptible to the majority of antifungal agents, apart from some copper-based products. Most bacterial plant pathogens are Gram-negative and/or produce abundant EPS which will tend to protect them from some antibacterial agents.

With annual plants, the aim is to reduce crop losses each season. With tree crops, there is the added problem that years of investment may be lost if a tree is killed or has to be destroyed in the interests of disease eradication. Even control by cutting out diseased parts can seriously affect the cropping of the tree for several years.

If food preservation principles could be followed, the solution would be to deprive the pathogen of water. The problem is how to do this without unduly depriving the host plant and hence reducing its yield. Temperatures can be manipulated in glasshouses but cooling is costly. Maintaining low soil nitrogen levels will also limit plant growth and crop yield and so can be counter-productive as a disease control measure.

For the present, approaches to disease control include: breeding for resistance; cultural measures and crop hygiene; use of chemical agents; and biological control. Integration of several methods is usually the best solution. A thorough understanding of the disease (including the influence of weather) is necessary if measures are to be applied to best advantage. There are few simple rules for control.

Resistance breeding

This is the most obvious solution to the problem of bacterial plant disease and has been successful in some cases but not in others. Useful resistance has been achieved in: alfalfa against *C. insidiosum*; cotton against *X. c. malvacearum*; tobacco, potato and tomato against *P. solanacearum*; and tomato against *C. m. michiganense*. Some crops have cultivars with useful degrees of resistance, even though they have not been bred for this purpose. In some losses may not be severe enough or sufficiently frequent to justify an extensive breeding programme.

A major problem with breeding for disease resistance is that a resistant plant may not be viable commercially either for cultural or for cropping reasons, or because the consumer or processor finds it unsatisfactory. With tree crops, resistance breeding is a slow process and success is rare. Where resistance involves only a few genes there is always the fear of a breakdown of resistance. Some resistance can break down when a plant is grown at higher temperatures than normal. Increased resistance to one disease may lead to increased susceptibility to another. Sometimes it has proved better to aim at reduction in susceptibility rather than a high level of resistance. It is possible that with new knowledge of the underlying mechanisms of pathogenicity plant breeding could be directed more precisely at a particular target in the host plant. New methods for producing resistant cultivars involving directed gene manipulation may be more successful. Breeding plants with tissue that it less susceptible to damage or to water-soaking could be one indirect approach.

Preventive measures

Some possible preventive measures are shown in Table 13 but they are a counsel of perfection and often fail. For commercial reasons and because of cryptic infections, diseased plants may be sold to the unwary. Where a disease appears in a new area, eradication rarely succeeds because the disease has often been present for

Table 13 Some preventive measures for limitation of bacterial plant diseases

Don't grow susceptible crops in climatic areas where disease risks are high
Don't introduce infected plants or seeds into areas where the disease has not yet appeared; quarantine 'healthy' plants introduced from infected areas
If a new disease appears, attempt eradication
Avoid susceptible cultivars, large plantings of single crops, susceptible alternative hosts
Avoid excessive manuring, leading to high soil nitrogen levels
Avoid tissue damage (especially during rain) from wind, insects, machinery, tools etc. and transfer of infection on tools
Avoid tissue water congestion through use of non-prone cultivars, shelter from wind-driven rain, good drainage, controlled irrigation, good glasshouse management
Destroy all infected plants and plant debris
Rotate crops where soil infestation is a problem
Understand the disease and use common sense

several seasons before it is detected. Eradication may succeed for a limited time in a limited area (as it did, for example, with citrus canker in Florida and fire blight in the Netherlands) but chances of reintroduction are high. Sometimes highly susceptible cultivars are the most desirable for commercial reasons and breeding for disease resistance does not always produce what a grower seeks. Sometimes alternative hosts are widespread as crops or wild plants and they cannot all be destroyed. Tissue damage is often difficult to avoid and frequent damaging storms may mean heavy losses in some climatic areas in some seasons. Infected plant material should probably be destroyed more often and more effectively than at present.

Comment so far suggests that failure is the rule but most of these measures succeed to some degree. One simple and effective measure is to grow seed crops in arid areas with controlled irrigation (not overhead) and seed potatoes in cool climates. Such measures can, however, break down in wet seasons. Prevention of cross infection during plant manipulations, including disinfection of tools, can prevent major losses in some instances. Common-sense measures can often prove valuable but if they are labour intensive may not be cost effective. A grower geared to spray programmes for control of other diseases and pests often wants an agent rather an a measure but this is not necessarily the best approach.

A novel preventive measure exists for blossom and leaf blights caused by frost damage due to the presence of ice-nucleating bacteria. The usual epiphytic bacterial population is replaced with bacteria which are identical, except that their ice-nucleating genes have been deleted. Deletion was simple, but obtaining permission to release genetically engineered bacteria outside the laboratory for field trials proved a major problem (Hirano and Upper, 1983; Lindow, 1983).

Chemical control

Many of the problems concerning the chemical control of bacterial plant diseases are discussed by Egli and Sturm (1980) and Jones in Mount and Lacey (1982). Suggestions for an ideal agent are shown in Table 14; this is a dream, not a reality. At present, antibiotics apart, the most successful agents for field use are copper-based compounds. Of these, Bordeaux mixture still seems to give the best control of fire

Table 14 Some requirements for an ideal agent for control of bacterial plant diseases

Desirable	Undesirable
Broad spectrum	Phytotoxicity
Systemic activity	Reduced crop yields
Tissue penetrating	Mammalian toxicity including carcinogenicity
Curative and protective	
Effective in the dormant period	Insect toxicity (pollinating insects)
Single application sufficient	Residues in edible crops
Control 95–100%	Incompatibility with other agents
Stable	Frequent applications necessary
Persistent	Persistence affected by weather
Easy to apply	Resistance development in the pathogen
Cheap; cost effective	

blight (*E. amylovora*) which is unfortunate because it needs to be freshly prepared and modern spray machines are not designed for its use. Other copper formulations (organic and inorganic) have proved useful with fire blight and other diseases but in all cases there is a danger of phytotoxicity. It seems that copper ions replace co-factors in vital plant enzymes or complex disruptively with plant carbohydrates and proteins; part of their effect may lie in hardening of plant surfaces, making tissue invasion more difficult. As an alternative to spraying, both antibiotics and copper sulphate have been injected under pressure into trees but this is still largely an experimental procedure.

The experimental agents, described by Egli and Sturm (1980), which have appeared most promising for control of bacterial plant disease are heterocyclic compounds containing nitrogen such as quinolene-3-carboxylic acids and related compounds. A therapeutic agent used in medicine, naladixic acid, which affects DNA synthesis of Gram-negative but not Gram-positive bacteria, belongs to this group. Some of these compounds have proved effective as protective agents in control of fire blight (*E. amylovora*) and others are effective against other *Erwinia* spp. None has yet been developed commercially for control of plant disease. Phenazine 5-oxide has proved useful for control of rice blight (*X. c. oryzae*); it interferes with biological redox systems.

Various other chemicals have been tried, including simple organic acids. Claims for success vary and it is often difficult to assess reports because essential details concerning inoculum levels, field factors and weather are lacking. It is success under high inoculum pressure and optimal environmental conditions for disease that matters and too often one or both of these factors are lacking in otherwise well-designed field trials. Adequate testing of new agents under field conditions can take many years because of wide fluctuations in the incidence and severity of most diseases.

With seed and tuber treatment, distinction has to be made between internal and external colonizers or contaminants. Hypochlorite can be useful for the latter. For bacteria within seeds, antibiotic solutions or slurries are sometimes used and also hot water treatment (but this may reduce germination and vigour). Success with any treatment is variable.

Disinfectants used for preventing cross-infection from tools include hypochlorite, phenolic-based compounds and ethanol. Sometimes undue faith is placed in disinfectants and the importance of contact time, poor penetration and reduction of activity in the presence of organic matter are not always appreciated.

Antibiotics

Limited use of medicinal antibiotics for plant disease control is permitted in the USA but not in most European countries, except for experimental purposes. Streptomycin has been used for control of fire blight (*E. amylovora*) on pear and apple trees since the 1950s. Streptomycin-resistant strains appeared in the 1970s (resistance seems to be chromosomal) and caused some growers to turn to oxytetracycline, much to the concern of many bacteriologists because of its widespread use in the treatment of human and animal disease. Unfortunately at present there are no alternative agents which are as cost effective and non-phytotoxic. Antibiotic resistance has also been reported in *X. c. vesicatoria* and *P. syringae*.

Biological control

Accelerated evolution (plant breeding) is one way to restore equilibrium in favour of the host plant; another way is to alter the epiphytic populations of bacteria in such a way as to prevent the pathogen from initiating disease. This is the basis for the control of crown gall and the prevention of frost damage by ice-nucleating bacteria. In the first case an isolate from natural sources is used; in the second, genetic manipulation is involved.

Details of the use of the K84 strain of *Agrobacterium* are described by Deacon in *Aspects* 7 (1983) and in other texts. K84 was isolated by Kerr and co-workers in Australia. Treatment is easy; cuttings or young, rooted plants are dipped in a suspension of the culture just before planting. This is not effective against all strains of the pathogen but disease prevention has been very successful in some cases. Strain K84 produces an adenine nucleotide analogue (trivial name Agrocin 84) which inhibits DNA synthesis—but it is only effective if the K84 population exceeds that of the pathogen at the infection site. The Ti-plasmid of *A. tumefaciens* codes for sensitivity to Agrocin 84 such that resistant strains are often (but not invariably) avirulent. Another twist in the story is that, as a result of recombination between an Agrocin producer and the pathogen, the pathogen may acquire the ability to produce the inhibitor and so become resistant to its action. Agrocin production in itself is not enough because the agent on its own is not effective; the whole bacterium is necessary. Competition for binding sites at the point of infection is suggested as the reason for this.

Success with *A. tumefaciens* stimulated hope that other pathogens might be controlled in similar ways, that is by finding a saprophytic bacterium that would become established at sites of infection and compete with the pathogen or produce antagonistic substances such as antibiotics, siderophores, bacteriocins and phages. There are, however, practical problems in applying this principle to major crops and major diseases where a simple dipping process is precluded. Also, for epiphytic bacteria to compete effectively with a pathogen, they usually have to be present in numbers that far exceed those of the pathogen. This is difficult to achieve under conditions favouring epidemic disease, and repeated sprays of bacterial suspensions to protect plants have serious disadvantages. Establishing alternative epiphytic bacterial populations may not be easy as they may have evolved to coexist with a particular plant but there are some encouraging examples of plant growth stimulation following introduction and of root-surface colonization by particular strains of bacteria, usually oxidase-positive *Pseudomonas* spp. This is a challenging field of study (Schroth and Hancock, 1981).

A difficulty with diseases affecting arial parts of plants is that the presence of the pathogen on the plant surface may be transient and too short for any antagonist to compete successfully. It seems unlikely that antagonistic bacteria would compete effectively with the pathogen once it has entered plant tissue. The target site for action would therefore seem to be the point of entry.

Progress in this area may not be rapid but it could well be the way in which novel approaches to disease control will emerge.

Storage rots

Control of rots in storage involves a variety of measures (Lund, 1983). These include minimimizing disease incidence in potato crops by using disease-free seed, good irrigation control, crop rotation and harvesting at the right stage of maturity; also, reducing numbers of the pathogen in the post-harvest environment by rapid disposal of plant debris, chlorination of washing and cooling waters and avoiding damage at all stages between harvesting and storage. Rapid cooling and optimum temperature, humidity and gaseous environment in the stores are also important. Crop losses from storage rots may exceed those from field diseases so prevention and control are of major importance.

Conclusion

There are no simple solutions to disease control. If the promise shown by recent work on underlying mechanisms of bacterial pathogenicity in plants is realized, then more rationally based control measures may emerge. Meanwhile, some possible strategies for control are suggested in Table 15.

Solutions often lie with the innovator who has the imagination to see alternative approaches or subtle variations on old themes. Sometimes this is someone with long experience gaining sudden insight; sometimes it is a complete outsider with a mind uncluttered with old solutions and an 'innocent eye'. Both are urgently

Table 15 Some possible strategies for control of bacterial plant diseases

Bacterial targets	Plant characteristics[a]
Growth rates	Encourage:
EPS	local cell death
Necrogenic ability	induced resistance
Pectic enzymes	high tissue calcium levels
Toxins	Increase rates of:
Ice-nucleating proteins	tissue maturation
Host specificity determinants	local tissue responses
High water requirements	walling off
Nutritional requirements	Decrease chances of:
Survival in tissue	damage
Dissemination factors	tissue water soaking
	succulent growth

[a] Some of these strategies might result in reduced crop yields.

needed in the field of bacterial plant disease control. But many seemingly promising projects from the past litter the highway. A prize for the control of fire blight offered in 1837 still awaits a claimant (van der Zwet and Keil, 1979).

Further reading

ALDWINCKLE, H. S. and BEER, S. V. (1979). Fire blight and its control. *Horticultural Reviews* 1: 423–74.

BILLING, E. (1984). Principles and applications of fireblight risk assessment systems. *Acta Horticulturae* 151: 15–22.

EGLI, T. and STURM, E. (1980). Bacterial plant diseases and their control. In: *Chemie der Pflanzenschutz und Schädlingsbekämfungsmittel*, Band 6 (edited by R. Wegler). Springer Verlag, Berlin, pp. 345–88.

HIRANO, S. S. and UPPER, C. D. (1983). Ecology and epidemiology of foliar bacterial plant pathogens. *Annual Review of Phytopathology* 21: 243–69.

LINDOW, S. E. (1983). The role of bacterial ice nucleation in frost injury to plants. *Annual Review of Phytopathology* 21: 363–84.

LUND, B. M. (1983). Bacterial spoilage. In: *Post-harvest Pathology of Fruits and Vegetables* (edited by C. Dennis). Academic Press, London and New York, pp. 219–257. (See also Lund in Mount and Lacey, 1982.)

PEROMBELON, M. C. M. and KELMAN, A. (1980). Ecology of the soft rot erwinias. *Annual Review of Phytopathology* 18: 361–87.

RUSSELL, G. E. (1978). Some examples of breeding for resistance to bacterial diseases. In: *Plant Breeding for Pest and Disease Resistance*. Butterworths, London, pp. 179–98.

SCHROTH, M. N. and HANCOCK, J. G. (1981). Selected topics in biological control. *Annual Review of Microbiology* 35: 453–76.

TENG, P. S. (1985). 'A comparison of simulation approaches to epidemic modelling. *Annual Review of Phytopathology* 23: 351–79.

THOMSON, S. V. (1986). The role of the stigma in fire blight infections. *Phytopathology* 76: 476–82.

VIDAVER, A. K. (1976). Prospects for control of phytopathogenic bacteria by bacteriophages and bacteriocians. *Annual Review of Phytopathology* 14: 451–65.

ZAUMEYER, W. J. (1932). Comparative pathological histology of three bacterial diseases of bean. *Journal of Agricultural Research* 44: 605–32.

VAN DER ZWET, T. and KEIL, H. L. (1979). *Fire Blight: A Bacterial Disease of Rosaceous Plants*. United States Department of Agriculture, Washington D. C.

7 Conclusions

At first sight, it would seem unlikely that plant pathogenic bacteria have much in common with those causing mammalian disease. However, among the Gram-negative opportunistic pathogens (*Pseudomonas* spp.), which produce a variety of tissue-damaging extracellular enzymes, some similarities are evident. In contrast there are no obvious parallels among mammalian pathogens with the macergenic *Erwinia* spp. or with *A. tumefaciens* but some of the necrogenic plant pathogens may have features that bear closer examination. Like many mammalian pathogens, though able to grow saprophytically on culture media, plant pathogenic bacteria are essentially host dependent. In the early stages of infection, damage to the host is limited but they may induce cell leakage. Bacterial capsules and EPS appear to have an important role and their loss leads to avirulence. Plant pathogens do not have to contend with an immune system and phagocytosis but, at the cellular level, there may be some parallels between phagocyte-bacterium and plant cell-bacterium interactions. The role of iron availability in plant disease remains to be determined.

At the simplest level, essentials for plant pathogenicity seem to be: the ability to transform plant cells to the advantage of the pathogen, or to produce pectic lyases under anaerobic conditions, or to multiply rapidly in intercellular spaces or in xylem vessels. Further there is a need to maintain a high water-potential in tissue without inducing plant stress reactions at an early stage. When more is known about the nature of interacting molecules in plants and pathogens, control measures might be more finely tuned to individual pathogens.

Medawar (1982) describes biology as 'complex, messy and richly various like real life' and the art of research as 'the art of making difficult problems soluble by devising means of getting at them'. There are now means of getting at some of the previously insoluble problems in plant pathology. Unfortunately there remain important ones that, for the present, are not soluble. The art is to distinguish between the soluble and the insoluble but still leave room for imagination so that future possibilities will not be missed.

Glossary

These outline definitions may sometimes prove inadequate outside the context of this book. Where they are explained in more detail in the book, page numbers are shown in parentheses. As an aid to further reading, some more complex terminology used in plant pathology is shown after the Glossary in Table 16.

Apoplasm: continuous space outside each living protoplast, including cell walls and free space (p.11).

Avirulent: applied to a variant of a pathogen no longer able to produce disease. See Chapter 5 and Table 16 for alternative use of this term.

Binding: joining; may be reversible (cf. Envelopment in cell-cell interactions).

Blight: widespread death of flowers, leaves and shoots.

Callose: a glucan formed in response to injury (p.44).

Callus: tissue formed in response to injury and in tissue culture (p.31).

Canker: sunken necrotic lesion of outer stem tissue.

Chlorosis: lack of normal green colour.

Commensal: sharing food with another organism without causing harm.

Compatible: able to coexist.

Complementary: able to combine (molecules).

Cortex: soft parenchymatous tissue located between the vascular system and the epidermis in plants (p.11).

Cultivar: a distinct subgroup (variety) of a plant species (p.51).

Elicitor: a molecule inducing the synthesis of phytoalexins from remote precursors (p.42).

Envelopment: bacteria surrounded by plant cell products; not necessarily immobilized.

Epiphytic: multiplying on plant surfaces without producing disease (p.62).

Fastidious: nutritionally exacting (p.5).

Gall: plant tumour (includes tissue, root and shoot proliferation).

Guttation: exudation of water and solutes through hydathodes.

Hydathode: water pore on leaf margin (p.35).

Hypersensitive reaction (HR): rapid localized plant cell and tissue death; characteristic of the interaction when an incompatible necrogenic pathogen is introduced into plant tissue.

Hypersensitivity: inflammatory immune response in mammals on second exposure to an antigen (cf. HR above).

Immobilization: bacterial growth and movement prevented following envelopment by plant cell products.

Incompatible: unable to co-exist.

Lenticel: air pore on outer surface of stem, root or tuber.

Lignin: phenylpropane polymers; confer rigidity in plants and resistance to degradation.

Macerate: a softened tissue in which cells have separated; a soft rot.

Macergenic: generating macerates; soft rotting (p.3).
Necrogenic: generating necrosis (cell death) (p.3).
Necrosis: death of cells or tissue (in plants, dead tissue often turns brown or black due to oxidation of phenolics).
Oncogenic: generating tumours (galls) (p.4).
Ooze: viscous fluid exuding from diseased plants; contains the pathogen surrounded by its own extracellular polysaccharide plus various plant products (p.25).
Opine: condensation product of an amino acid and a keto acid (p.33).
Opportunistic pathogen: saprophyte which takes advantage of lowered host resistance.
Parenchyma cells: generally thin-walled, relatively undifferentiated.
Pathogenic: able to cause disease.
Pathovar: strain of a species with distinctive pathogenicity to one or more host plants (p.7).
Phloem: nutrient-conducting tissue, notably for sugars (p.11).
Phytoalexin: a low-molecular-weight antimicrobial agent commonly produced by a plant in response to infection and injury (p.42).
Phytotoxic: toxic to plants.
Plasmadesmata: pores in cell walls connecting protoplasts of adjoining cells (see Symplasm) (p.11).
Race: a distinct subgroup of a pathogenic species or pathovar (p.51).
Receptor: sensitive to a distinct (specific) signal molecule.
Recognition: discrimination between molecules or pathogens (p.38).
Repress: prevent (e.g. signal-receptor interaction).
Resistance: relative capacity to resist infection (c.f. Susceptibility).
Resistant: able to prevent infection by a particular pathogen (c.f. Susceptible).
Saprophyte: living on dead tissue.
Signal: a molecule initiating an interaction when combined with a specific receptor (p.38).
Specific: distinct, unique.
Stomata: air pores on leaves (p.35).
Suberin: waxy, hydrophobic deposit.
Susceptibility: relative dispostion to infection.
Susceptible: unable to prevent infection by a particular pathogen (c.f. Resistant).
Symplasm: continuous space within the plant body which is enclosed by the plasma membrane and connected by plasmadesmata (c.f. Apoplasm) (p.11).
Systemic: moving through the plant.
Tonoplast: membrane enclosing the vacuole in the cytoplasm of the plant cell.
Virulence: relative capacity to cause disease.
Virulent: fully pathogenic; able to produce all the typical symptoms of the disease in a susceptible host (c.f. Avirulent). See Chapter 5 and Table 16 for alternative use of this term.
Xylem: water-conducting tissue (p.11).

Table 16 Some terminology comparisons

Terms used in this book	Terms sometimes used in plant pathology
Pathogen[a]	
Wide host-range pathogen	Non-specialized pathogen
Narrow host-range pathogen	Specialized pathogen
Virulent strain	Pathogenic strain/isolate
Avirulent strain	Non-pathogenic strain/isolate
Compatible race	Virulent race
Incompatible race	Avirulent race
Incompatibility gene	Avirulence gene
Plant[b]	
Non-host	General resistance
Heterologous host resistance	Race non-specific resistance (horizontal)
Cultivar resistance	Host resistance
Homologous host resistance	Race-specific resistance (vertical)
Plant-pathogen interaction[a, b]	
Compatibility (species-species)	General/basic compatibility
Compatibility (cultivar-race)	Specific compatibility
Incompatibility (species-species) leading to HR	Non-specific recognition leading to a general resistance reaction (HR)
Incompatibility (cultivar-race) leading to HR	Specific recognition leading to a specific resistance reaction

[a] With pathogens, host specificity may lie at the species, pathovar or race level.
[b] With plants, the susceptible group may be at the species, supraspecies or subspecies level.

Abbreviations

CWDE: cell wall degrading enzymes
EPS: extracellular polysaccharides
FP: fastidious prokaryotes
HR: hypersensitive reaction
HRGP: hydroxyproline-rich glycoproteins
IAA: indole acetic acid
LPS: lipopolysaccharide
MLO: mycoplasma-like organisms
RLB: rickettsia-like bacteria

C. m.: *Corynebacterium michiganense*
E. c.: *Erwinia carotovora*
P. s.: *Pseudomonas syringae*
X. c.: *Xanthomonas campestris*

pv, pvs: pathovar(s).
sp., spp.: species(s)

Bibliography

Multiple-author texts

Useful sources of further reading in addition to those listed at the end of each chapter are listed here.

CALLOW, J. A. (ed.) (1983). *Biochemical Plant Pathology*. John Wiley & Sons, Chichester.

CIVEROLO, E. L., COLLMER, A., DAVIS, R. E. and GILLASPIE, A. G. (eds) (1987). *Plant Pathogenic Bacteria*. Proceedings of the Sixth International Conference on Plant Pathogenic Bacteria. Martinus Nijhoff, Dordrecht.

DAY, P. R. and JELLIS, G. J. (eds) (1986). *Genetics and Plant Pathogenesis*. Blackwell Scientific Publications Ltd, Oxford.

DENNIS, C. (ed) (1983). *Post-Harvest Pathology of Fruits and Vegetables*. Academic Press, London.

FAHY, P. C. and PERSLEY, G. J. (eds) (1983). *Plant Bacterial Diseases: A Diagnostic Guide*. Academic Press, Sydney.

GOULD, G. W., RHODES-ROBERTS, M. E., CHARNLEY, A. K., COOPER, R. M. and BOARD, R. G. (eds) (1986). *Natural Antimicrobial Systems*. Bath University Press, Bath.

INGRAM, D. S. and WILLIAMS, P. H. (eds) (1982). *Advances in Plant Pathology*, Vol. 1. Academic Press, London.

KOSUGE, T. and NESTER, E. W. (eds) (1984). *Plant-Microbe Interactions*. Macmillan Publishing Co., New York.

MOUNT, M. S. and LACEY, G. H. (eds) (1982). *Phytopathogenic Prokaryotes*, Vols 1 and 2. Academic Press, New York.

RHODES-ROBERTS, M. E. and SKINNER, F. A. (eds) (1982). *Bacteria and Plants*. Academic Press, London.

ROBERTS, K., JOHNSTON, A. W. B., LLOYD, C. W., SHAW, P. and WOOLHOUSE, H. W. (eds) (1985). *The Cell Surface in Plant Growth and Development*, Suppl. 2, *Journal of Cell Science*. The Company of Biologists Ltd, Cambridge.

See also titles in the series *Aspects of Microbiology* edited by J. A. Cole, C. J. Knowles and D. Schlessinger including:

1. Oral microbiology (2nd edn). P. D. Marsh and M. V. Martin (1984).
2. Bacterial toxins (2nd edn). J. Stephen and R. A. Pietrowski (1986).
4. Bacterial plasmids (2nd edn). K. Hardy (1986).
6. Bacterial cell structure. H. J. Rogers (1983).
7. Microbial control of plant pests and diseases. J. W. Deacon (1983).
9. Extracellular enzymes. F. G. Priest (1984).

Handbooks and practical guides

AGRIOS, G. N. (1978). *Plant Pathology*, 2nd edn. Academic Press, New York.
BRADBURY, J. F. (1986). *Guide to Plant Pathogenic Bacteria*. Commonwealth Agricultural Bureaux, Kew, Surrey.
GERHARDT, P. (ed.) (1981). *Manual of Methods for General Microbiology*. American Society for Microbiology, Washington D. C.
GOODMAN, R. N., KIRALY, Z. and WOOD, K. R. (1986). *The Biochemistry and Physiology of Plant Diseases*. University of Missouri Press, Columbia, Missouri.
KRIEG, N. R. and HOLT, J. G. (1984). *Bergey's Manual of Systematic Bacteriology*, 9th edn, Vol. 1. Williams & Wilkins, Baltimore.
LELLIOTT, R. A. (1986). Viruses and bacteria. In: *Handbook of European Plant Diseases*, Vol. 1. Blackwell Scientific Publications Ltd, Oxford.
LELLIOTT, R. A. and STEAD, D. E. (1986). *Methods for Diagnosis of Bacterial Diseases of Plants*. Blackwell Scientific Publications Ltd, Oxford.
MAZZUCHI, U. (1981). *Elementi di Bateriologia Fitopatologica*, Vols 1 and 2. Pitagora Editrice, Bologna.
MEDAWAR, P. (1982). *Pluto's Republic* (incorporating *The Art of the Soluble* and *Induction and Intuition in Scientific Thought*). Oxford University Press, Oxford.
MEYNELL. G. G. and MEYNELL, E. (1970). *Theory and Practice in Experimental Bacteriology*, 2nd edn. Cambridge University Press, Cambridge.
ROITT, I. M., BROSTOFF, J. and MALE, D. K. (1985). *Immunology*. Churchill Livingstone, Edinburgh.
SMITH, E. F. (1905, 1911, 1914). *Bacteria in Relation to Plant Disease*, Vol 1,2 and 3. Carnegie Institute, Washington D. C.
SNEATH, P. H. A. (ed.) (1986). *Bergey's Manual of Systematic Bacteriology*, 9th edn, Vol. 2: Williams & Wilkins, Baltimore.
STARR, M. P. (ed.) (1982). Phytopathogenic bacteria. In: *The Prokaryotes: A Handbook of Habitats, Isolation and Identification of Bacteria* (edited by M. P. Starr, H. Stolp, H. G. Trüper, A. Balows and H. G. Schlegel, Springer Verlag, New York.
SUTHERLAND, I. W. (ed.) (1977). *Surface Carbohydrates of the Prokaryotic Cell*. Academic Press, London.

Advisory Leaflets published by the Ministry of Agriculture, Fisheries and Food in England, and similar publications produced in other countries, provide valuable information on individual diseases.

Index of Bacteria

Subject Index